A HISTORY

OF THE

DISCOVERY

OF THE

CIRCULATION OF THE BLOOD,

BY P. FLOURENS;

Perpetual Secretary of the Academy of Sciences, (Institute of France ;) Member of the Royal Societies and Academies of Science of London, Edinburgh, Stockholm, Munich, Turin, Madrid, Brussels, etc., etc. Professor at the Museum of Natural History of Paris.

Etant sur les bancs, il fit une action d'une audace signalée, qui ne pouvait guère, en ce temps-là, être entreprise que par un jeune homme, ni justifiée que par un grand succès; il soutint dans une thèse la circulation du sang. Les vieux docteurs trouvèrent qu'il avait défendu avec esprit cet étrange paradoxe.—FONTENELLE, *Eloge de Fagon.*

TRANSLATED FROM THE FRENCH,

BY J. C. REEVE, M. D.

CINCINNATI:
RICKEY, MALLORY & COMPANY.
1859.

TRANSLATOR'S PREFACE.

A desire for information in regard to the history of a science, as naturally follows its study as does the wish to know something of the countries through which we travel, or of the biography of authors whose works have instructed or amused us. To medical men the satisfaction of this desire is attended with something more than the mere gratification of curiosity; lessons of great practical value are to be derived from the study of the history of medicine. As we observe the slow and uncertain manner in which our present knowledge has been attained, we shall feel that our progress is likely also to be gradual, and that the great discoveries of the future are to be made, like those of the past, by patient and long continued observation, judicious experiment and careful generalization. As we see the doctrines of great teachers, which were received by their followers as infallible, shown one after the other to be erroneous, we may learn caution in regard to resting our efforts with the present attainments of science. For these and many other reasons the study of the history of medicine is valuable to the practitioner, and has always been recommended to the student, by those best qualified to judge, as an important part of his professional education.

There are, however, few books upon medical history accessible to readers in this country. The voluminous work of Sprengel has never been translated into the English language. The excellent History of the Inductive Sciences by Whewell is but partially occupied with medical subjects, and, until the appearance of Prof. Comegys' translation of Renouard's History of Medicine, the profession has been limited to the brief sketch upon this subject by Dr. Bostock in the Cyclopedia of Practical Medicine.

From the condensed form necessary, when so wide a subject as the history of medicine is considered within the limits of an essay or even of a single volume, the discovery of the circulation of the blood does not receive that attention which it merits, either in the article by Dr. Bostock or in the work of Renouard. This discovery may be said without exaggeration, to be one of the most important events in the history of medical science; some of the greatest minds ever in the profession took part in it; it exerted an important influence upon the treatment of disease, it marked a new era in the history of medicine, and effected a revolution in scientific research. All who reflect upon these facts will be convinced that it deserves a separate treatise.

This little work of M. Flourens has been translated and is now presented to the profession of this country in hopes that it may help to supply information upon a most important part of medical history. If after availing himself of the literary resources of the French capital, the author found the history of this discovery imperfect, it is surely unnecessary to apologize for offering in this country the result of his efforts to complete it. The faithfulness and ability with which he has performed his task are guaranteed by his attainments and his position; as a scientific man and as an eminent medical writer, he has so long been known to the world, as to render any introduction here superfluous.

Dayton, Ohio, May, 1859.

AUTHOR'S PREFACE.

Some years ago, while looking over Ramazzini's *Commentaire* upon Cornaro, my attention was arrested by the following paragraph:

"The ancients were entirely ignorant of the circulation of the blood, and we are indebted to Harvey, the English Democritus, for making it known, after having derived it from those two excellent sources, Fabricius ab Aquapendente and Paul Sarpi, both professors at Padua, and who made so many experiments upon all sorts of animals."

This paragraph awakened my curiosity; I made research; I found writers partizan, biased, and prejudiced; of the true historian, the judge, I could not find a trace. The history of the discovery of the circulation of the blood was yet to be written.

I study successively in this work all the wonderful discoveries of the circulation of the blood properly speaking, of the lacteals, of the reservoir of the chyle, and of the lymphatics. I follow the facts from Erasistratus and Galen to Servetus, from Servetus and Cæsalpinus to Harvey, from Harvey to Pecquet and Thomas Bartholin.

One point has particularly occupied my attention, I have applied myself to the investigation, and, if I may so speak, to the reconstruction of all the ideas of Galen in regard to the circulation in the adult and in the fœtus, the formation of the blood and of the *spirits*, and the origin of animal heat.

In one chapter are examined the pretensions of Sarpi to the discovery of the circulation of the blood, and in another the physiological doctrines of Servetus, that strange man of genius! I close with two chapters upon Guy-Patin, the most obstinate and at the same time most talented adversary which modern doctrines encountered.

HISTORY OF THE DISCOVERY

OF THE

CIRCULATION OF THE BLOOD.

I.

HARVEY AND THE CIRCULATION OF THE BLOOD.

The discovery of the circulation of the blood did not belong, and could scarcely belong to a single man, nor indeed to a single age. Many errors were to be destroyed; in place of these errors truths were to be established; and this was accomplished slowly, little by little. Galen commenced the discovery by combatting Erasistratus; he opened the route which followed afterward by Vesalius, by Servetus, by Columbus, by Cæsalpinus and by Fabricius ab Aquapendente conducted us to Harvey.

Three principal errors masked, if I may so speak, the great fact of the circulation of the blood. The first was, that the arteries contained only air; the second, that the septum, between the two ventricles of the heart, was perforated; and the third, that the veins carried the blood to the extremities instead of bringing it from them.

Let us see with whom these errors originated and who destroyed them.

Erasistratus.

Erasistratus held that the arteries contain air; he did not believe that they contain blood.

According to him the air drawn by the lungs penetrated to them by the trachea (*trachée artere*); from the trachea it passed into the *venous artery* (which we now call the pulmonary vein,) from thence it entered the left ventricle, passed on into the arteries and was distributed by them to the system at large.[1]

What we now call the sanguineous system, the circulating system, was then divided into two—the *arterial* or *œrian* and the *venous* or *sanguineous* system.

The arteries were ærian canals, or channels for air; hence their name of *arteries*, and hence their similarity of name to the *trachée artere*, which is the great air-passage of the body.

(1) According to Erasistratus we respire only to fill the arteries with air. "Quænam est utilitas respirationis? ...... Num animæ ipsius generatio est? ...... An innati caloris ventilatio ac refrigeratio? .... Aut horem quidem nihil est, verum arteriarum expletionis gratiâ respiramus, velut Erasistratus putat?"—(*De utilitate respirationis, Galeni opera, edition des Junte. Venise*, 1597, p. 223.)

Galen.

As soon as an artery is opened, says Galen, the blood gushes out of it: then one of two things must be true, it was either contained in the artery or came into it from elsewhere. But, if the latter, if the artery contained nothing but air, the air should come out before the blood, and this does not take place; blood alone comes out and no air; then the arteries contain nothing but blood.[1]

Galen made another experiment. He placed two ligatures on an artery a little distance apart; he opened the canal between them and found nothing but blood: once more then, the arteries contain blood and they contain nothing but blood.[2]

But, cried the followers of Erasistratus, if the arteries contain blood, how can the air which is drawn in by the lungs pass into all parts of the

(1) Quoniam arteriâ quâcumque vulneratâ, sanguinem egredi videmus, duorum alterum sit oportet, vel in arteriis sanguinem contineri, vel aliunde ipsum in eas confluere. Quod, si aliunde sanguis in eas confluit, manifestum est unicuique, cum se naturaliter arteriæ habebant, spiritum ipsas solummodo continuisse. Quod, si hoc verum esset, oportebat in vulneratis, priusquam sanguis egrederetur, spiritum exire conspiceremus; cum autem hoc fieri non videamus, nec anteà solum spiritum in arteriis contentum fuisse colligemus.—(*An sanguis in arteriis naturâ contineatur*, p. 60.)

(2) Ubi funiculo dissectam arteriam utrinque ligavimus, et quod in medio comprehensum fuerat incidimus, sanguine plenam ipsam esse monstravimus.—(*Ibid.* p. 61.)

body? It does not pass there, responded Galen: the air which is drawn in is rejected again; it serves for respiration by its *temperature* and not by its *substance;* it *cools* the blood and that is the end and aim of respiration.[1]

Assuredly this is very far from what we now know of the respiration. It is even directly contrary to what takes place. Instead of *cooling* the blood, respiration *heats* it; respiration is the source of *animal heat;* but yet, compared with the doctrines of Erasistratus, who held that the air passed into the arteries in totality, *en masse*, in substance, as it passes into the trachea and into the bronchiæ, that it was the air which filled the arteries, which distended them,[2] and made them beat, that it was

(1) Sed quomodo, reclamant, in totum corpus aer veniet, quem respirando attrahimus, si sanguineum arteriæ contineant? Quibus respondendum est, quæ necessitas hoc eos fateri cogat, cum possit totus, qui respirando admissus est aer, foras esse remitti: quemadmodum pluribus, iisque diligentissimis tam philosophis quam medicis, visum est, qui cor, inquiunt, non aeris substantium exposcere, sed frigiditatem solummodo, quâ recreari desiderat: atque hunc esse respirationis usum.—(*Ibid.*, p. 62.)

(2) .... "Consentiens Erasistrati sententiæ; quandoquidem putat arterias. ...... ideo distendi, quod compleantur spiritu (the spirit, that is to say, for Erasistratus, the *air;* it will be seen farther on what Galen considered the *spirit*), à corde suppeditato."—(*De pulsuum differentiis*, p. 69.)

the air which caused the pulse,[1] the idea of Galen was a progress, and such a progress that physiology was not able to advance beyond it until she called to her aid the resources of modern chemistry. Haller believed still that respiration *cooled* the blood.

Thus then it was established that the arteries do not contain air; they contain only blood like the veins; an entire half of the sanguineous system, which had been detached by an hypothesis, was given back to it again; and, as the circulation is but the unceasing movement of the blood from the heart into the arteries, and from the arteries into the veins, and through the veins back again to the heart, so long as the arteries were supposed to contain nothing but air the discovery of the circulation was impossible: without the first step which Galen made it was impossible to make a second.

Of the three principal errors, then, first mentioned, there was one less; one was destroyed. But Galen was not so happy with the two others. He still believed that the septum between the two ventricles was perforated, and that the veins carried the blood to the extremities: two errors which were destined to pass from him to the moderns, and the latter of which is opposed to the very idea of the circulation.

(1) "Pulsus est dilatatio arteriæ, quæ completione fit spiritus à corde emissi."—(*Ibid.*)

The first modern anatomists.

The septum which separates the two ventricles is not perforated. How did it happen then that Galen believed it to be perforated—*saw* it thus? Because he imagined it necessary that it should be so!

According to Galen the veins, as well as the arteries, carried blood to the extremities; but according to him there were two kinds of blood—the *spiritual blood*, the blood of the arteries and of the left ventricle, and the *venous blood*, the blood properly speaking, the blood of the veins and of the right side of the heart.[1] And this was another step in advance. It was the first indication of the two kinds of blood now so well distinguished, the red blood and the black blood,—the arterial and the venous blood,—the blood which has, and that which has not been purified by respiration.

There were then, according to Galen, two kinds of blood; and each kind had a destination peculiar to itself: the *spiritual blood* nourished organs of light and delicate texture, such as the lungs; the *venous blood* nourished those heavy and gross, such as the liver.[2] The *spirit*, the *purest part of the*

(1) .... Sinistro ventriculo, quem medici *spirituosum* appellare consueverunt .... altero ventriculo, quem *sanguineum* appellant.—(*De usu partium*, lib. vi, p. 150.)

(2) Ut similem, ad sui nutritionem, postulent sanguinem, verbi gratiâ hepar viscerum omnium gravissimum ac densis-

blood,[1] was only formed in the left ventricle;[2] it being necessary, however, that even the *venous blood* should contain a certain proportion of *spirit*[3] in order to fit it for the purposes of nutrition, it was also necessary that the two ventricles, the ventricle of the spirit and the ventricle of the blood, should communicate with each other, and this communication was held to take place by means of foraminæ in the septum which separated them.[4]

Galen, therefore, held the septum to be perforated because he had imagined a system which rendered a communication between the ventricles necessary. The early modern anatomists believed the septum perforated because Galen had said it was so!

simum, et pulmo levissimus ac rarissimus .... Quo factum est ut hepar quidem à venis fere solis, ... pulmo vero ab arteriis nutriretur.—(*Ibid.*, p. 155.)

(1) Spiritus exhalatio quædam est sanguinis benigni ...... (*Ibid.*)

(2) Spiritus receptaculum, sinister ventriculus .... (*De anat. administ.*, lib. vii., p. 95.)

(3) Demonstratum nobis alio loco est, omnia esse in omnibus ....; atque arteriæ quidem tenuem ac purum et vaporosum participant sanguinem, venæ autem paucum, eumdemque caliginosum aerem .... (*De usu partium*, lib. vi., p. 154.)

(4) Quæ igitur in corde apparent foramina, ad ipsius potissimum medium septum, prædictæ communitatis gratiâ, extiterunt.—(*Ibid.*, p. 155.)

Mondini said the septum was perforated;[1] Vasseus, or Le Vasseur, to whom I shall refer again, said the same as Mondini;[2] twenty others made the same statement. Berenger de Carpi first avowed that these openings *were only to be seen with difficulty;*[3] and Vesalius, the great Vesalius, the father of modern anatomy, Vesalius alone dared say that *they did not exist.* He did not, however, arrive at that point directly. He commenced by repeating, like all the others, that the blood passed from one ventricle to the other through *openings in the septum.*[4] But soon, carried away by the force of the truth which he saw, the fact which he

(1) He calls the septum the *middle ventricle:* Nam iste ventriculus non est una concavitas, sed plures concavitates parvæ, ... ut sanguis qui vadit ad ventriculum sinistrum à dextro, cum debeat fieri spiritus, continuo subtilletur ...... —(*Anatomia Mundini.* Ed. of Dryander, 1540, p. 38.)

(2) "Within the heart there are two sinuses or ventricles separated by a partition, called in Latin *septum,* through the openings in which the spirit and the blood have communication."—(*French translation, by Canappe,* p. 46.)

(3) In homine cum maximâ difficultate videntur.—(*Commentaria super Anat. Mundini,* p. 341, ed. 1521.) Sylvius, or Dubois, also did not seem willing to admit the foraminæ of the septum; at least he does not speak of them; he contents himself with saying—Sunt cordi ventres duo, carnis ipsius portione mediâ, ceu diaphragmate quodam secreti.—(Ed. 1555.)

(4) .... Maximâ portione per ventriculorum cordis septi poros in sinistrum ventriculum desudare sinit .... (*Vesalii Opera Omnia Anatomica,* ed. d'Albinus, 1725, t. i., p. 517.)

touched, he declared that he only made that statement in order *to accommodate himself to the teachings of Galen;*[1] for, in truth, the structure of the septum is no less solid or compact than the rest of the heart, and through this dense tissue there can not pass a single drop of blood.[2]

Galen showed that the arteries contain blood as well as the veins, and this was the first step; he pointed out the distinction between the two kinds of blood, the *arterial* and the *venous*, and this was the indication of a second step; Vesalius had just shown that the partition between the two ventricles is not perforated and this was the third step; one step more and the pulmonary circulation was discovered. This step was made by Servetus.

Servetus and the pulmonary circulation.

I shall carefully guard against making any allusion to the theological works of Servetus, which I

(1) In cordis constructionis ratione, ipsiusque partium usu recensendis, magnâ ex parte Galeni dogmatibus sermonem accommodavi.—(*Ibid.*, p. 519.)

(2) Haud levitur studiosis expendendum est ventriculorum cordis interstitium, aut septum, ipsumve sinistri ventriculi dextrum latus, quod æque crassum, compactumque ac densum est, atque reliqua cordis pars sinistrum ventriculum complectens, adeo ut ignorem .... quì per septi illius substantiam ex dextro ventriculo in sinistrum vel minimum quid sanguinis assumi possit.—(*Ibid.*, p. 519.)

have never read.[1] Perhaps in his quarrels with Calvin he was as much at fault as his adversary, but, at least, he did not burn Calvin.

I shall confine myself to the following passage upon the *pulmonary circulation*, and I maintain that this admirable passage alone is sufficient to give to its author an illustrious place among men of science.

The communication, says Servetus, (that is to say, the passage of the blood from the right to the left ventricle,) does not take place through the median partition of the ventricles, as is generally supposed; but by a long and wonderful route the blood is conducted through the lungs, where it is agitated and prepared, where it becomes yellow, and passes from the arterial vein into the venous artery: *et à venâ arteriosâ in arteriam venosam transfunditur.*

I stop a moment at these words, *et à venâ arteriosâ in arteriam venosam transfunditur*, for they express the new and complete idea.

Even while supposing the inter-ventricular septum to be perforated Galen knew very well that the blood of the right ventricle passed, at least in part, through the pulmonary artery into the lungs.[2]

(1) I have had occasion to read some of them since this was written as will be seen farther on.

(2) Atqui orificia omnia sunt numero quatuor, duo in utroque ventriculo: in sinistro unum quod spiritum de pulmone

Vesalius was also aware of it.[1] But this was only the half of the truth.

The entire and complete idea necessary to establish the pulmonary circulation was to understand that the blood passed from the *pulmonary artery* into the *pulmonary veins;* that the blood leaving the right heart by the pulmonary artery, returned to the left heart by the pulmonary veins; that the blood left the heart and returned to the heart; that there was, consequently, a *circuit, circulation;* and this idea of the *circulation,* so grand and so new, was first formed by Servetus.

In order to understand how this communication takes place by the lungs, said Servetus, we must *learn* the connection, the multitude of unions of the *arterial vein* with the *venous artery* in this

immittit, alterum quod educit: reliqua duo in dextro, alterum quod in pulmonem sanguinem emittit alterum quod è jecore admittit.—(*De Hipp. et Plat. decret.*, lib. vi., p. 264.)

(1) Dexter ventriculus .... a cava venâ, quoties cor dilatatur ac distenditur, magnum sanguinis vim attrahit, quem, adjuvantibus forte ad hoc ventriculi foveis, excoquit: ac suo calore attenuans, levioremque, et qui aptius impetu postmodum per arterias ferri possit reddens, maximâ portione per ventriculorum cordis septi poros in sinistrum ventriculum desudare sinit (it is seen on page 19 that he admitted these *openings* in the *septum* only out of complaisance to Galen), reliquam autem ejus sanguinis partem, dum cor contrahitur arctaturque, per venam arterialem in pulmonem delegat.—(*Vesalii, Op. omnia anat.* Ed. 1725, t. i., p. 517.)

organ. And this view of the manner of communication is confirmed by the calibre of the *arterial vein*, which would not be so large, nor carry such an amount of blood to the lung, if nutrition alone was to be provided for, especially since in the embryo (and this is an exceedingly ingenious remark,) the lung is nourished through other channels and this blood does not reach it. It must be then for another purpose that the blood is sent in such abundance from the heart to the lungs immediately after birth. It is sent there to be mixed with air, for it is not air alone, but air mixed with blood, that passes into the venous artery. The yellow color is given to the blood by the lungs and not by the heart.[1]

(1) Fit autem communicatio hæc non per parietem cordis medium, ut vulgò creditur, sed magno artificio à dextro cordis ventriculo, longo per pulmones ductu, agitatur sanguis subtilis; à pulmonibus præparatur; flavus efficitur, et a venâ arteriosâ in arteriam venosam transfunditur.—(*Christianismi Restitutio:* Totius Ecclesiæ apostolicæ ad sua limina vocatio, in integrum restitutæ cognitione Dei, fidei Christi, justificationis nostræ, regenerationis baptismi et cœnæ Domini manducationis; restitutio denique nobis regno cœlesti, Babylonis impiæ captivitate solutâ, et Antichristo cum suis penitus destructo.—*Viennæ Allobrogum*, MDLIII.)

[In an appendix to the work of M. Flourens are some ten or twelve pages, being all the physiological parts, of this singular work of Servetus, so interesting in the history both of physiology and of theology. As full extracts are made

All this is full of sagacity, acuteness and penetration. The connection or union of the pulmonary artery with the pulmonary vein in the lungs by an infinite number of branches; the calibre of the pulmonary artery, which would be much too large if it served only for the nutrition of the lungs; the nutrition of this organ in the embryo without the blood of the pulmonary artery, which indeed does not then transmit any; all these are most excellent and decisive reasons—the same which we give now— the true ones.

Let us remark again upon the change of color in the blood which takes place not in the heart, but in the lung, and is due to the action of the air. We know now that it is not the whole of the air which produces this change, but the oxygen alone. But except that, except the analysis of the air, which has been the work of modern chemistry, how near these ideas were to the truth! Servetus not only discovered the true route of the blood from one side of the heart to the other through the lungs; he also discovered the true place of

concerning the author's discovery of the pulmonary circulation, and his peculiar views are fully explained in the text, it has not been deemed necessary to re-print here that additional amount of matter not so immediately connected with the subject. All the quotations from Servetus which follow are taken from the work, the title of which is given above in full.—*Tr.*]

sanguification, of the *transformation* of the blood, of its change from black blood to red. Galen placed the seat of sanguification in the liver; Servetus first located it in the lungs; a truth which was not then remarked, which was not comprehended until long afterward, and which indeed did not receive its full development until very recent times by the experiments of Goodwin and Bichat.[1]

The passage of the blood from one ventricle into the other, continues Servetus, is not through the septum; in the same manner that the blood of the *vena porta* passes into the *vena cava* through the liver, so the blood of the *arterial vein* passes into the *venous artery* through the lungs.[2]

(1) Quod ita per pulmones fiat communicatio et præparatio docet conjunctio varia et communicatio venæ arterio-sæ cum arteriá venosá in pulmonibus. Confirmat hoc magnitudo insignis venæ arteriosæ, quæ nec talis, nec tanta facta esset, nec tantam à corde ipso vim purissimi sanguinis in pulmones emitteret, ob solum eorum nutrimentum, nec cor pulmonibus hâc ratione serviret, quum præsertim anteà in embryone solerent pulmones ipsi aliunde nutriri... Ergo ad alium usum effunditur sanguis à corde in pulmones horâ ipsâ nativitatis, et tam copiosus. Item à pulmonibus ad cor non simplex aer, sed mixtus sanguine mittitur per arterium venosam. Ergo in pulmonibus fit mixtio. Flavus ille color à pulmonibus datur sanguini spirituoso, non à corde.

(2) Demum paries ille medius, quum sit vasorum et facultatum expers, non est aptus ad communicationem et elabora-

A nearer approach to the truth could not have been made without finding it. Finally, said Servetus in closing, and he could safely say it, if any one will compare these things with what Galen has written in the sixth and seventh books of his work, *De usu partium*, he will see clearly the truth which Galen did not perceive.[1]

Columbus.

Six years after Servetus, Realdo Columbus, one of the best anatomists Padua ever had, (Padua which had so many of them; Vesalius, Columbus, Fallopius, Fabricius ab Aquapendente!) Realdo Columbus discovered again and independently [2] the *pulmonary circulation.*

Between the two ventricles, said he, is the septum through which it is believed the blood passes

tionem illam... Eodem artificio, quo in hepate fit transfusio à venâ portâ ad venam cavam propter sanguinem, fit etiam in pulmone transfusio à venâ arteriosâ ad arteriam venosam propter spiritum (or more exactly, propter *sanguinem spirituosum.*)

(1) Si quis hæc conferat cum iis quæ scribit Galenus, lib. vi et vii. *De usu partium*, veritatem penitus intelliget, ab ipso Galeno non animadversam.

(2) See in chap. iv what is said farther upon this point. Neither Columbus, nor those who came immediately after him could have been acquainted with the work of Servetus.

from the right to the left; but this is a great mistake, for the blood is carried by the *arterial vein* into the lungs; from thence it passes, with the air, by the *venous artery* into the left ventricle of the heart, which no one has yet seen: *quod nemo hactenus aut animadvertit, aut scriptum reliquit, licet maxime sit ab omnibus animadvertendum.*[1]

Cæsalpinus.

Finally, Cæsalpinus described in his turn, and without citing Columbus, (whom he surely did not know, since he does not allude to him: great merit is always honest,) the *pulmonary circulation;* and this time not merely the fact appears but also the word. Cæsalpinus formally named the passage of the blood from one side of the heart to the other by the lungs, the *circulation.*

This *circulation,* said he, which carries the blood from the right heart through the lung into the left, corresponds perfectly with the disposition of the

(1) Inter hos ventriculos septum adest, per quod fere omnes existimant sanguini à dextro ventriculo ad sinistrum aditum patefieri; ... sed longâ errant viâ: nam sanguis per arteriosam venam ad pulmonem fertur, ibique attenuatur; deinde cum aere unà per arteriam venalem ad sinistrum cordis ventriculum defartur: quod nemo hactenus aut animadvertit, aut scriptum reliquit, licet maxime sit ab omnibus animadvertendum. (Realdi Columbi, *De re anatomicâ,* edition 1572, p. 325.)

parts. For each ventricle has two vessels, one by which the blood arrives and the other by which it departs; the vessel by which the blood arrives at the right ventricle is the *vena cava*, that by which it leaves is the *pulmonary artery;* the vessels which pour the blood into the left ventricle are the *pulmonary veins*, the vessel which affords it exit is the *aorta.*[1]

Thus then was the *pulmonary circulation* discovered.

Cæsalpinus and the general circulation.

The pulmonary circulation was discovered; but so far, until Cæsalpinus, not a word had been uttered in regard to the *general circulation*, the circulation of the body, which we call the *greater* in comparison to the pulmonary which we term the *lesser*.

(1) Huic sanguinis *circulationi* ex dextro cordis ventriculo per pulmones in sinistrum ejusdem ventriculum optime respondent ea quæ ex dissectione apparent. Nam duo sunt vasa in dextrum ventriculum desinentia, duo etiam in sinistrum. Duorum autem unum intromittit tantum, alterum educit, membranis eo ingenio constitutis. Vas igitur intromittens vena est magna quidem in dextro, quæ cava appellatur; parva autem in sinistro ex pulmone introducens.... Vas autem educens arteria est magna quidem in sinistro, quæ aorta appellatur, parva autem in dextro, adpulmones derivans... (Andreæ Cœsalpini, *Quæstionum peripateticarum*, lib. v, p. 125, édition des Junte. Venise, 1593.)

Galen originated a very symmetrical physiology. According to him there were four temperaments, the *sanguine*, the *phlegmatic*, the *bilious*, and the *atra-bilious;* and four humors, *blood*, *phlegm*, *bile*, and *black bile;* he had also three kinds of *spirits*, the *natural*, the *vital*, the *animal;* and three sources of these spirits, the *liver*, the *heart* and the *brain!*

Farther, the *brain* was the origin of all the *nerves*, the *heart* of all the *arteries*, and the *liver* of all the *veins*.

The veins, having their source in the *liver*, carried the blood to all parts of the body. Strange error! one that the most simple experiment, or even the most simple attention to an occurrence coming under daily observation, would have served to destroy. For certainly bleeding was practiced every day, and every day the vein must have been seen to swell *below* and not *above* the ligature, showing that the course of the blood in the veins was from the extremities to the heart, and not from the heart to the extremities.

There is an excellent chapter in Vesalius on the utility of experiments on living animals. Vesalius truly remarks, that a simple experiment on a living animal will teach more than long observation of the dead body. For instance, if one wishes to know whether the arteries contain blood or air, it is only necessary to open an artery in a living animal, and it is seen that it contains blood.[1] Unhappily Vesalius stopped with the *arteries;* he did not pass on to the veins ; he was content to believe, in regard to them, that a simple inspection of the dead animal sufficed "to show that they carried the blood to the extremities."[2]

Cæsalpinus was the first, and the only one before Harvey, who called attention to the swelling of the veins which takes place *below* and never *above* the ligature. It is a very curious thing, he observes, that the veins become distended below the ligature and not above it. Those who bleed patients, added he, are familiar with the fact; they always place the ligature *above* the place of puncture and not *below* it: *quaia tument venæ ultrâ vinculum non citrâ;* which should be just the contrary if the movement of the blood was from the heart toward the external parts of the body.[3]

(1) Atquæ ita levi negotio observatur in arteriis sanguinem naturâ contineri, si quando arteriam in vivis aperimus. —(*Ibid*, p. 568.)

(2) Cæterum in venarum usu inquirendo, vix quoque vivorum sectione opus est: quum in mortuis affatim discamus eas sanguinem per universum corpus deferre.—*Ibid*, p. 568.

(3) Sed illud speculatione dignum videtur, propter quid ex vinculo intumescunt venæ ultrà locum apprehensum, non citrà: quod experimento sciunt qui venam secant; vincu-

He says elsewhere: the blood conducted to the heart by the veins, receives there its perfection, and this perfection acquired, it is carried by the arteries to all parts of the body.[1] A better conception of the general circulation could not be found, nor a better definition be given in as short a sentence.

Cæsalpinus possessed a mind of a superior order. He was the first among the moderns, who fully appreciated *method* in classification, or classification founded upon organism..[2] Before his time plants were classified according to their external appearances, their names, supposed medicinal virtues, etc. In the *classification of plants* by Cæsalpinus, all the characteristics are drawn from the plants themselves; and guided by a happy tact, he recognised first the most important organs and those which furnish the most important characteristics, the organs of fructification, the flowers,

lum enim adhibent citrà locum sectionis, non ultrà; quia tument venæ ultrà vinculum non citrà. Debuisset autem opposito modo contingere, si motus sanguinis et spiritus à visceribus fit in totum corpus... (*Quæstionum medicarum*, lib. ii, same edition, p. 234.)

(1) In animalibus videmus alimentum per venas duci ad cor tanquam ad officinam caloris insiti, et, adeptâ inibi ultimâ perfectione, per arterias in universum corpus distribui, agente spiritu, qui ex eodem alimento in corde gignitur. (*De plantis*, Florence, 1583, lib. ii, cap. II, p. 3.)

(2) ["Method is the soul of science."—*Linnæus*.]

fruits and grains. Cæsalpinus has the double glory of having been the first to give us a *method* in science, and the first to point out the *two circulations.*

Fabricius ab Acquapendente.

Fabricius ab Acquapendente has also two honors; he discovered the *valves* of the veins, and he was the teacher of Harvey.

Fabricius discovered the valves of the veins in 1574. He saw well that they open toward the heart. They oppose, therefore, any passage of the blood from the heart to the external parts in the *veins;* it must go then from the parts toward the heart—the reverse of what takes place in the *arteries,* which have no valves.

The valves of the veins are the anatomical proof of the circulation of the blood—the proof that it makes a circuit, that it returns upon itself, that it *circulates.* But Fabricius did not understand this proof; he saw the fact, but failed to draw from it that important deduction which was left for the genius of Harvey.

Sarpi.

Something should here be said of Sarpi, to whom has been attributed both the discovery of the circulation of the blood and of the valves of the veins.

As to the discovery of the circulation, his claim is founded upon a paper discovered among his manuscripts after his death by Father Fulgence. In this paper we are assured that Sarpi describes the circulation of the blood.

In regard to the valves, Gassendi relates in his Life of Peiresc, that Peiresc told him that the discovery of the valves of the veins was due to Sarpi, who confided it to Fabricius.[1] But Fabricius tells us positively that he discovered the valves of the veins himself. They were, says he, unknown before the year 1574, when I perceived them for the first time with great joy; *summâ cum letitiâ.*[2]

Fabricius was a man of surpassing knowledge in anatomy, and as respectable morally as he was intellectually; and he quotes Sarpi elsewhere in regard to some observations he had made upon the action of light on the pupil.[3] But we are forced to conclude, with Tiraboschi, that although Sarpi

(1) De quibus (*valvulis*) ipse aliquid inaudierat ab Acquapendente, et quarum inventorem primum Sarpium Servitam meminerat.—(*Vita Peyreschii*, lib. iv., p. 222.)

(2) De his itaque in præsentiâ locuturis, subit primum mirari quo modo ostiola hæc ad hanc usque ætatem tam priscos quam recentiores anatomicos adeo latuerint, ut non solum nulla prorsus mentio de ipsis facta sit, sed neque aliquis prius hæc viderit quam anno 1574, quo à me summâ cum lætitiâ inter dissecandum observata fuere.—(*De venarum Ostiolis: Hieronymi Fabrici ab Acquapendente Opera omnia anatomica.* Edition d'Albinus, 1737, p. 150.)

(3) De oculo, visus organo.—(Same edition, p. 229. The quotation will be found farther on.)

may possibly have taken part in the discovery of the circulation of the blood, more and other proof of the fact must be furnished, before it can be considered established.[1]

Vasseus or Le Vasseur, and a quotation of M. Portal.

Le Vasseur was a disciple of Jacques Sylvius or Dubois, who was first the master and the very worthy master of Vesalius, and afterward the fiercest of his adversaries.

Le Vasseur wrote a small work in Latin, which was little if any thing more than an abridgment of the anatomy and physiology of Galen. This little work passed through several editions, and from the first, was translated into French by *maître Jean Canappe, docteur en médecine.*

M. Portal, in his *Histoire de l'anatomie,* says that Le Vasseur "knew almost as much as we do of the circulation of the blood." "For fear," adds he, "that I may be accused of having mutilated the text I will give the author's own words:

Dextrum ventriculum, qui sanguineus appellatur, vena cava ingreditur, et vena arteriosa egreditur quæ in pulmonem dispergitur, sanguinem elaboratum conferens. . . . . Sinistro ventriculo cordis qui

(1) Io dunque non negherò al Sarpi l'onor di questa scoperta, ma bramerò solamente che se ne possan produrre più certe et più autentiche pruove.—(*Storia della letteratura italiana,* t. vii., p. 597.)

caloris nativi fons est, et spirituosus appellatur, arteria venosa quæ ex pulmone . . . . M. Portal stops at these words, *quæ ex pulmone*, and the reader, following the impulse which has been given completes the sentence; *which brings the blood back again from the lungs to the heart;* and consequently Le Vasseur "knew as much as we do of the circulation." But not at all! Le Vasseur was not speaking of the *blood*, he was speaking of *air!*

Here is the entire paragraph which I give from the old French of Canappe:

"The vena cava empties into the right ventricle which is called sanguineous, and from which departs the arterial vein which is dispersed and distributed to the lung and carries the elaborated blood . . . . Into the left ventricle, which is the fountain of natural heat, and is called spiritus, is inserted the venous artery, which brings from the lung, (and it is at this word that Portal stops) which brings from the lung air to the heart, and evacuates from here the fuliginous excrements."

Harvey.

When Harvey appeared every thing relative to the circulation of the blood had been indicated or suspected; nothing had been established. Nothing had been established; and this is so true that Fabricius, who comes after Cæsalpinus, and who discovered the valves of the veins, knew nothing of the circulation.[1] Cæsalpinus himself who so plainly perceived the two circulations, mixed with the idea of the pulmonary circulation the error of a perforated septum. *Sanguis partim per medium septum, partim per medios pulmones . . . . ex dextro in sinistrum ventriculum cordis transmittitur.*[2] Servetus said nothing of the general circulation. Columbus repeated, after Galen, the fictions of the origin of the veins in the liver[3] and the transmission of blood to the extremities by them.[4]

I admit, with Sprengel, that nothing explains Harvey better than "*his education at Padua.*"[5]

(1) He believed that the only use of the valves was to prevent too great an accumulation of blood in the inferior parts of the body, an occurrence which would be attended with the double inconvenience of too great a supply to the lower parts and too small a quantity in the upper. Eâ ratione, uti opinor à naturâ genitæ, ut sanguinem quadamtenus remorentur, ne confertim, ac fluminis instar, aut ad pedes, aut in manus et digitos universus influat, colligaturque; duoque incommoda eveniant, tum ut superiores artuum partes alimenti penuriâ laborent, tum vero manus et pedes tumore perpetuo premantur.—(*Loc. cit.*, p. 150.)

(2) *Quæst. peripatet.*—(Lib. v., p. 126.)

(3) Est igitur jecur omnium venarum caput, fons, origo et radix, p. 300.

(4) Venæ nihil aliud sunt quam vasa concava .... ut sanguinem ad singula membra deferant fabrefacta, p. 305,

(5) Sprengel's History of Medicine, French translation by Jourdan. Paris, 1815, tom. iv., p. 87.

Undoubtedly this education at Padua was a piece of good fortune for Harvey, but it was also, if I may be allowed so to express myself, a piece of good fortune for the circulation to pass into the hands of Harvey, the man most capable of studying it, of investigating it, of comprehending it in all its relations, and of placing it in its true light before the world.

Harvey has been reproached for not citing his predecessors; but he quotes Fabricius who discovered the valves without perceiving their uses;[1] he cited Columbus who had most strongly combatted the error of the perforated septum;[2] finally he

(1) Clarissimus Hieronymus Fabricius ab Acquapendente, peritissimus anatomicus et venerabilis senex, ... primus in venis membraneas valvulus delineavit, figurâ sigmoides, vel semilunares portiunculas tunicæ interioris venarum, eminentes et tenuissimas .... Harum valvularum usum inventor non est assecutus, nec alii addiderunt; non est enim ne pondere deorsum sanguis in inferiora totus ruat: sunt namque in jugularibus deorsum spectantes, et sanguinem sursum prohibentes ferri: nam ubique spectant à radicibus venarum versus cordis locum .... (Gulielmi Harvei *Exercitatio anatomica de motu cordis et sanguinis*, cap. xiii.)

(2) Cur non iisdem argumentis, de transitu sanguinis in adultis per pulmones, fidem similem habent, et cum Columbo, peritissimo, doctissimoque anatomico, idem asserunt, et credunt ex amplitudine, et fabricâ vasorum pulmonum? Arteria enim venosa, et similiter ventriculus, repleti sunt semper sanguine, quem venis huc venisse necesse est, nullâ aliâ quam per pulmones semitâ, ut et ille, et nos ex ante dictis et autopsiâ, aliisque argumentis palam esse existimamus.—(Cap. vii.)

came from Padua where the state of the question was fully understood, where every thing which had been said upon the circulation was known by all.

Harvey's work is a master-piece. This little book of a hundred pages is the most beautiful volume on physiology. Harvey commenced with the movements of the heart; and first, he remarked that the auricle and the ventricle of each side of the heart contract successively. When the right auricle contracts, the blood passes into the right ventricle; when the right ventricle contracts, the blood passes into the pulmonary artery; from the pulmonary artery it passes into the pulmonary veins; from thence it goes into the left auricle which contracts and forces it into the left ventricle, the contractions of this ventricle expel it through the aorta into all the arteries of the body and from them it is collected by the veins and returned to the heart from whence it started. At each passage from one cavity into another he observed there were valves, membranes, little gates, (*ostiola*, as Fabricius calls them), which open to allow the blood to pass one way and close to prevent its passage in the opposite direction. The valves of the right auricle allow the blood to pass into the ventricle but prevent its return into the auricle; the valves of the ventricle allow it to pass into the pulmonary artery but prevent it from coming back into itself; on the left side the valves of the auricle allow its passage into the ventricle but not backward, and those of the ventricle permit its onward course into the aorta and in no other direction; the valves of the veins present no obstruction to its course toward the heart but bar its passage back toward the arteries.

After the heart, came the arteries. Galen attributed the pulsations of the arteries to a *pulsific virtue*, which they derived from the heart with their tunics. He made an experiment to prove this statement, but he made it badly. He opened an artery and introduced a tube through the opening; he then tied the artery over the tube and as he tied it too tightly the blood ceased to flow, or flowed only in very feeble jets; the artery ceased to beat below the ligature and Galen concluded, therefore, that the beating of the arteries depended upon a *pulsific virtue* drawn by their coats from the heart, since a simple ligature sufficed to prevent the pulsation in all that part of the artery on its distal side.[1]

(1) Arteriam unam è magnis et conspicuis quampiam, si voles, nudabis; primoque pelle remotâ ipsam ab adjacenti suppositoque corpore tamdiu separare non graveris quoad filum circum immittere valeas; deinde secundum longitudinem arteriam incide, calamumque et concavum et pervium in foramen intrude, vel æneam aliquam fistulam, quo et vulnus obturetur, et sanguis exilire non possit. Quoadusque sic se arteriam habere conspicies, ipsam totam pulsare videbis: cum primum vero obductum filum in laqueum contrahens ar-

Harvey did not repeat the experiment of Galen. It is too complicated, and he believed it scarcely possible.[1] He contented himself with more simple observations. He saw that when an artery was opened the blood came out in unequal jets, alternately stronger and feebler; he observed that the stronger jets always corresponded with the *diastole* of the artery and not with the *systole;* he concluded that it was the impulse, the shock of the blood which distended the artery and caused it to beat. If the artery dilated of its own inherent power it could not expel the blood with the greatest force at the moment of greatest dilatation.[2]

Harvey profited farther by a case of *ossification* of the femoral artery which came under his obser-

teriæ tunicas calamo obstrinxeris, non amplius arteriam ultrà laqueum pulsare videbis, etiamsi spiritus et sanguis ad arteriam, quæ est ultrà filum, sicuti prius faciebat, per concavitatem calami feratur; quod si propterea pulsabant arteriæ, pulsarent nunc partes quæ sunt ultrà laqueum, sed non pulsant: igitur perspicuum est, quum moveri posse desinunt, non propter spiritum in concavitatibus discurrentem, sed ob virtutem in tunicas transmissam, arterias à corde moveri.—(*An sanguis in arteriis naturâ contineatur*, p. 62.)

(1) Nec ego feci experimentum Galeni, nec recte posse fieri vivo corpore ob impetuosi sanguinis ex arteriâ eruptionem puto .... (*Prœmium.*)

(2) .... Sed et in arteriotomiâ et vulneribus contrarium manifestum est. Sanguis enim saliendo ab arteriis profunditur cum impetu, modo longius, modo propius vicissim prosiliendo, et saltus semper est in arteriæ diastole et non in

vation; the artery pulsated *below* the ossification; the ossification did not prevent the transmission of the pretended *pulsific virtue*, or rather no such virtue existed; the arterial pulsation is only due then to the movement of the blood,—solely to the impulse of the blood against the walls of the artery.[1]

systole. Quo clare apparet impulsu sanguinis arteriam distendi. Ipsa enim dum distenditur, non potest sanguinem tantâ vi projicere .... (*Ibid.*)

(1) Sed quo clarius, quod in dubio est appareat, pulsificum vim non per arteriarum tunicas a corde manare, habeo, e nobilissimi veri cadavere, arteriæ descendentes portionem, cum duobus cruralibus ramis, spithamæ longitudine, exemtam, in os fistulosum conversam; per cujus cavum, dum vivebat nobilissimus vir, descendens arteriosus sanguis in pedes subditas arterias suo impulsu agitabat; in quo tamen casu arteria idem passa, tanquam si super canaliculum fistulosum constricta et ligata foret (secundem Galeni experimentum) ut neque dilatari, eo loco, neque arctari ut follis, neque vim pulsificam a corde inferioribus et subditis arteriis communicare, aut per soliditatum ossis deducere facultatum, quam non susceperat, potuerit. Nihilominus inferioris arteriæ pulsum agitari in cruribus et pedibus optime menimi, dum vivebat, me sæpissime observasse .... Quare in illo nobilissimo viro necesse inferiores arterias ab impulsu sanguinis, ut *utres*, dilatatas fuisse, non ut *folles* ab expansione tunicarum.—(*Exercitatio altero ad J. Riolanum.*) But this is not all. I have repeated the experiment of Galen; far from being *scarcely possible* as Harvey believed, it is not even very difficult. I have opened the aorta of a sheep and introduced a quill, I have tied the artery over this tube and have seen the blood continue to pour out through it (which certainly did not take place in Galen's experiment, or at least only partially, either on ac-

From the arteries Harvey passed to the veins; and it is from their valves that he drew the important deduction to which I have already alluded, viz: that they allow to the blood but one course, movement only in the direction toward which the valves open, a movement from the external parts of the body toward the heart.

Finally Harvey made his experiments; they were few but decisive, and in this is shown his genius.

When a ligature is tied lightly around an extremity the blood is arrested in the veins alone because they alone are superficial; when the ligature is tied tightly the blood is also stopped in the arteries which lie deeper.

When a vein is tied the swelling takes place *below* the ligature; when an artery is tied it takes place *above;* the blood then flows in directly opposite directions in the arteries and veins; it flows from the extremities to the heart in the latter, and from the heart to the extremities in the former.[1]

count of the ligature having been too tight or because the tube became obstructed); the blood continued to flow and the artery continued to beat *below* as well as *above* the ligature. The *pulsative faculty* of Galen is not then wholly imaginary. The blood distends the artery, and because it is distended it pulsates. (See experiments upon the pulsations or movements of the arteries, in my *Recherches experimentales sur les propriétés et les fonctions du systeme nerveux;* Paris, 1842.

(1) In my lectures at the *Jardin des Plantes*, I make the following experiment, under the eyes of my pupils, to illustrate

When any artery whatever is opened, and the blood allowed to flow freely, all the blood of the body is lost through this opening; then all parts of the circulating system communicate with one another, heart, arteries, and veins.

A moment's reflection, in truth, upon the marvelous rapidity of the movement of the blood will convince one that it must necessarily be thus; for scarcely has the blood arrived at the heart when it leaves it and enters the arteries, no sooner has it entered them than it commences to pass into the veins, and from the veins it goes immediately into the heart again; this course, this continual *return* is the *circulation.*

Modern physiology dates from the discovery of the circulation of the blood. This discovery marked the entrance of the moderns into science. Until then they had followed the ancients; they dared now walk alone. Harvey had discovered the most beautiful phenomenon of the animal economy; one to which all antiquity had never been able to arrive. What became then of the authority of the masters? Authority was dethroned; it was no longer neces-

the circulation of the blood. I cause the crural vein and artery of a dead dog to be opened; a tube is inserted into the open end of the artery and water is injected by means of a syringe; in a few minutes the water injected into the artery runs out of the vein. It is a complete illustration of the cir culation.

sary to swear by Galen and by Aristotle, but by Harvey.

I will relate, farther on, the ridiculous obstinacy with which the faculty rejected the circulation; the bad reasonings of Riolan, the unhappy pleasantries of Guy Patin. But this wrong belonged only to the faculty, not to the nation. Moliere ridiculed Guy Patin, and Boileau ridiculed the faculty.[1] Before Moliere and Boileau the greatest of moderns, Descartes, had proclaimed the circulation: "But if it be demanded how the blood in the veins is not exhausted by this perpetual flow into the heart, and how the arteries are not filled to overflowing, since all that goes into the heart is poured into them, I have only to give as an answer that which has been written by a physician of England, to whom we must give the honor of having first investigated this subject, and of being the first to teach that there are at the extremities of the arteries many little passages through which the blood received from the heart passes into the small branches of the veins, and through these vessels returns to the heart; so that its course is nothing but a perpetual circulation."[2]

After Descartes we must quote Dionis.

While the faculty was rejecting the circulation

(1) See *l'Arret burlesque.*

(2) *Discours de la méthode.* Ed. of M. Cousin, p. 179.

Dionis taught it in the *Jardin du Roi.* "I was chosen to demonstrate in your royal garden," says Dionis in his dedication to Louis XIV., "the circulation of the blood and the new discoveries, and I acquitted myself of this duty with all the ardor and the exactitude which the orders of your Majesty deserve." These words honor the memory of Louis XIV.

Thus upon one side France devoted a chair to the teaching of the circulation of the blood, and on the other, as we shall soon see, completed this great work by the discovery of the reservoir of the chyle (*receptaculum chili*) by Jean Pecquet.

So far I have exhibited what belongs to Harvey in the discovery of the circulation of the blood, but I have only spoken of the circulation in the adult; it remains to be seen how much he contributed toward the discovery of the *fœtal circulation.*. This will be the subject of the following chapter.

II.

DUVERNEY AND THE FŒTAL CIRCULATION.

The heart of the fœtus is not like that of the adult. In the adult the two sides of the heart are completely separated. An entire and solid membrane, like that between the ventricles, separates the two auricles, and the two large arteries, the pulmonary artery and the aorta, have no communication with each other.

In the fœtus all this is different. The septum between the two auricles is perforated by an opening called the *foramen ovale* and the pulmonary artery and aorta are connected by a canal which we call the *ductus arteriosus.*

What are the objects of this conformation?

First, let us remark that there are two points to examine—structure and use. Galen was acquainted with the structure; Harvey discovered the use.

Galen.

In the fœtus, says Galen, the *vena cava* opens into the *venous* (pulmonary) *artery.*[1] The *arterial vein* and the *grand artery* (pulmonary artery and

(1) "In fœtibus vena cava in arteriam venosam est pertusa."—(*De usu partium,* lib. xv., p. 212.)

aorta) are likewise united by a third vessel which nature has formed expressly for that purpose.[1] And as the two first-named vessels, the vena cava and the pulmonary artery, touch each other, nature has made an opening from one to the other, and has applied a membrane to this opening, which yields readily to the blood as it passes from the vena cava to the venous artery, and resists on the contrary, the return of the blood from the venous artery back into the vena cava.[2]

All this is admirable, adds Galen; but what is still more admirable is that a few days after birth, this opening between the vena cava and the venous artery closes; the canal which unites the arterial vein and the great artery becomes obliterated; and he who would seek for these early communications some time later will not be able to find them; of one of them, of the opening between the vena

(1) "Verum cum hæc vasa inter se aliquantum distarent, aliud tertium vas exiguum, quod utrumque conjungeret, natura efficit."—(*De usu partium.*)

(2) "In reliquis vero duobus, cum hæc mutuo sese contingerent, velut foramen quoddam utrique commune pertudit: tum membranam quamdam in eo, instar operculi, est machinata, quæ ad pulmonis vas facile resupinaretur, quo sanguini à venâ cavâ cum impetu affluenti cederet quidem, prohiberet autem ne sanguis rursum in venam cavam reverteretur."—(*Ibid.*)

cava and the venous artery he will not find a trace.[1]

It must not be supposed, continues Galen, that we are speaking of communications or openings small, scarcely visible, and doubtful; the openings are large, evident, patent, of which there can be no question; their existence has been denied however, but to those who are unbelieving I will say, if they have eyes I will convince them, if they have no eyes, if they are blind, they at least have hands and I will make them touch them.[2]

(1) "Hæc quidem omnia naturæ opera sunt admiranda: superat vero omnem admirationem prædicti foraminis, haud ita multo post, conglutinatio. Etenim, quamprimum animans in lucem est editum, ... membranam, quæ est ad foramen, coalescentem reperias, nondum tamen coaluisse; cum autem animal perfectum fuerit, ætateque jam floruerit, si locum hunc ad unguem densatum inspexeris, negabis fuisse aliquando tempus in quo fuerit pertusus......... Pari modo id vas, quod magnam arteriam venæ quæ fertur ad pulmonem connectit, cum aliæ omnes animalis particulæ augeantur, non modo non augetur, verum etiam tenuis semper effici conspicitur, adeo ut, tempore procedente, penitus tabescat, atque exsiccetur."—(*De usu partium.*)

(2) .... Et ego iis, qui nos ita insectantur, si modo oculos habent, ostentam magnæ arteriæ propaginem, et venæ cavæ orificium, ... sin vero sunt cæci, vasa in manus sibi imposita contrectare jubebo; nam neque exiguum eorum utrumque, neque vulgare est, sed amplum admodum, commemorabilemque intra sese habet meatum, quem non solum is qui oculos habet non ignoraverit, sed ne is quidem cui tangendi erit potestas, si solum ad anatomen velit accedere."—(*Ibid.*)

The anatomists of the time of Galen strongly resembled the anatomists of all times, ever slow to observe and ever ready to accuse those who observed of being deceived. Galen compared them to the man who, in counting his asses, forgot the one upon which he was mounted and immediately accused his neighbors of having stolen one! They were like this man because in the enumeration of errors they always forgot those of which they themselves were guilty.

The early modern anatomists; Vesalius and Fallopius.

Among modern anatomists Fallopius was the first to see the *ductus arteriosus*, and Vesalius the first to observe the *foramen ovale*. These two great men had frequent occasion to encounter each other;[1] they created modern anatomy; they possessed the spirit of investigation in the highest degree, and both were men of most superior mind.

Fallopius, commenting on Vesalius, is astonished that this *portion of canal*, or *artery*, which unites the *arterial vein* with the *aorta*, could so long have escaped the attention of anatomists—and consequently of Vesalius; especially as in the fœtus the canal is widely open, and although obliterated afterward, it still remains as a thick, hard body;

(1) Vesalius wrote an *Examination of the Observations* of Fallopius, and the *Observations* of Fallopius are in fact a continual examination of the *Anatomy* of Vesalius.

and finally Galen has spoken of it, although certainly in but few words: *verbis paucissimis tamen.*[1]

You are astonished, writes Vesalius in reply, that anatomists make no mention of a canal which unites the *arterial vein* and the *great artery;* and, upon this subject, you quote a passage of Galen, taken from Book xv. of *De usu partium.* My dear Fallopius, this passage did not escape me, and much less that of Book vi., which I wonder extremely you do not remember, in which Galen, as well as in the passage of Book xv., speaks not only of this communication, but of another placed between the *venous artery* and the *vena cava.*[2]

Vesalius admits, in another place, that not having paid sufficient attention to the great vessels,

(1) "In arteriarum historiâ illud in memoriam venit, quod non levem admirationem excitat: 1. quâ ratione factum sit, quod anatomici fere omnes tam negligenter observarint partem illam canalis vel arteriæ, quâ jungitur vena arterialis circa basim cordis ipsi aortæ; cum in fœtu tam aperta pateat, tantusque sit aditus ab aortâ ad venam arterialem ...... Secundo quia à Galeno in decimo quinto *De usu partium,* cap. sexto, aliquot (paucissimis tamen) verbis designatur."—(Gabrielis Faloppii *Observationes anatomicæ:* in the edition of the *Œuvres de Vesale,* already quoted, t. ii., p. 730.)

(2) "Cæterum (ut ad te redeam) miraris plurimum anatomicos nullam fecisse mentionem unionis mutuæque apertionis venæ arterealis ad magnam arteriam, Galenique locum ex decimo quinto *De usu partium* adducis. Mi Fallopi, hic locus me non latuit, ac multo minus is, cujus miror hic te non meminisse, et quo in sexto *De usu partium,* Galenus, perinde

the *ductus arteriosus* had escaped his observation. But, since, he had turned to the examination of the heart of the fœtus, and immediately the *foramen ovale* presented itself to him.[1] He mentions the oval form of this opening: *ovatâ prœditum effigie.* He studied the *ductus arteriosus;* he opened it;[2] and with his attention fixed upon the passage of Galen,[3] he admires the clearness with which that great man had described it: *miratus fui quamobrem Galenus hic tam dilucide vasis privatim meminit, quo vena arterialis in magnam arteriam pertinet.*

Arantius and Carcanus.

Arantius was the pupil of Vesalius; Carcanus was the student of Fallopius. No sooner had Ve-

ac in decimo quinto, non tantum hanc unionem, verum et illam, quæ arteriæ venali cum cavâ venâ obtigit, satis prolix et (si quis animum sedulò intendit) aperte commemorat."—(Andreæ Vasalii *Opera*, t. ii., p. 798.)

(1) At quum propagines quasdam, ut veluti vasa quædam ex uno vase in aliud producta, extra magnorum vasorum cavitates parum recte pervestigarem, illam unionem non reperi .... Mox in fœtu, venæ cavæ caudicem, ... longâ sectione secundum rectitudinem aperui. Hic sese tum nihil manifestius mihi obtulit quam maximum venæ cavæ in venalem arteriam pertinens foramen."—(t. ii., p. 798.)

(2) "Pari artificio, venæ arterialis caudicem .... longâ etiam sectione patefeci, caudicisque illius cum magnâ arteriâ unionem et mutuum foramen observavi."—(*Ibid.*)

(3) "Sedulo Galeni locis rursus perlectis."—(*Ibid.*)

salius and Fallopius laid with so much *eclat*, the foundations of the anatomy of the adult, than their pupils began to investigate the anatomy of the fœtus.

Arantius, in his work on the *human fœtus*, commences by informing us that he only proposes to make more clear what Galen has so well written on the vessels and heart of the fœtus.[1] Carcanus expresses himself in the same manner.[2]

Here then, it will be said, was a very remarkable concord in rendering homage. Vesalius and Fallopius disputing as to who could proclaim most loudly the discovery of Galen; Arantius and Carcanus partaking this great admiration and continuing the praise.

Assuredly if after this a desire to name either of these things seized anatomists, the *foramen ovale* for instance, it would receive the name of Galen, and be called *foramen Galeno.* But not at all— it is called the *foramen Botalli!*

(1) "Quod cordis vasa, aorta scilicet venæ arteriali, et vena cava arteriæ venali, conjugantur, Galenus optime declaravit. .... sed cum ab ipso non ita perspicuè despripta fuerint, ut facile à minus exercitatis intelligi possent, ad ejus sententiæ explicationem pauca quædam addere constitui."—(*De humano fœtu*, edition of 1595, p. 37.)

(2) *De vasorum cordis in fœtu unione.*

Botal.

Botal was not strictly an anatomist. He was a bold physician, who arriving in Paris[1] at a time when the faculty abused purgatives, could scarcely fail of making an impression, for he abused blood-letting.[2] The faculty purged their patients without mercy, and he bled his without pity. The faculty became angry.[3] Botal persevered; from Botal to Broussais those who have held out against the faculty have soon become celebrated.

Botal, in dissecting a subject one day, found, what sometimes happens in adult life, the foramen ovale open; he saw it and immediately imagined that he had made the greatest discovery which could be made !

Some time ago, says he, when reflecting upon the discord between Galen and Columbus in regard to the route which the blood follows in passing through the heart, Galen maintaining that it passes by foraminæ in the median septum, and Columbus by the venous artery, I opened a heart and immediately perceived a very large conduit, leading directly from the right auricle into the left, which conduit, or vein, can by good right be named the *nutritive vein of the arteries*, for through

(1) Botal was from Asti, in Piedmont.

(2) See his treatise *De curatione per sanguinis missionem.*

(3) Much was written upon blood-letting on both sides, and the controversy was extremely beneficial.

it the *arterial blood* passes into the left ventricle, and from there goes into all the arteries, and it does not pass through the *septum*, or by the *venous artery*, as Galen and Columbus have believed.[1]

Botal was here mistaken on every point! first, the blood which passes through the foramen ovale from the right into the left auricle is not *arterial* blood, but *venous*, the pretended *vein* could not possibly then be called the *nutritive vein of the arteries:* second, this opening does not exist in the adult, or only exists as an exception, it is a peculiarity of fœtal existence, and this, of all who have written upon it, Botal alone did not comprehend; and finally, Botal tells us that the opening or conduit (*vein*, as he calls it,) had not been observed

(1) Diebus iis proxime peractis, cum Galenum atque Columbum dissentire viderem de viâ, quâ in cor sanguis, qui per arterias vagatur, fertur, asserente Galeno hunc in cor transfundi per parva foraminula cordis septo insita, Columbo vero per alia (Columbus did not say *per alia*, but *per arteriosam venam*, and he said rightly. Botal did not perceive how important exactitude was. See Chap. I.) ad arteriam venosam,...cor dividere occœpi, ubi...satis conspicuum reperi ductum, juxtà auriculam dextram, qui statim in sinistram aurem recto tramite fertur; qui ductus, vel vena, jure arteriarum...... nutrix dici potest, ob id quod per hanc feratur *sanguis arterialis* in cordis sinistrum ventriculum, et consequenter in omnes arterias, non autem per septum, vel venosam arteriam, ut Galenus vel Columbus putaverunt., (Botalli *Opera omnia*, edition of Van Horne, 1660, p 66.)

by any one previous to him; *a nullo anteâ notata*:[1] yet the *foramen ovale* had been seen and described, and admirably described, by Galen, by Vesalius, by Arantius and by Carcanus!

The uses of the ductus arteriosus and foramen ovale.

Galen asks himself what can be the use of the *ductus arteriosus* and of the *foramen ovale*, and responds to his own inquiry.

But his answer is wholly theoretical; it is extremely complicated and finely drawn, yet in every point coherent, which is the mark of a great master. Galen can not be explained in portions; in studying his theories the great whole must be kept in view or nothing will be understood.

Here, for example, the idea he has of the uses of the *ductus arteriosus* and the *foramen ovale* agrees with those concerning the veins and arteries; his ideas of the veins and arteries agree with those in regard to the two species of blood, the *spirituous* blood and the *venous* blood; and the idea which he had framed of these two kinds of blood are in harmony with his conceptions of the nature of organs, of which some require more of the *spirituous* blood than of the *venous* and others exactly the reverse.

(1) "*Vena arterianum nutrix, à nullo anteà notata*:" such is the title under which Botal published his pretended discovery.

The lungs require more of the *spirituous* than of the *venous blood:* all the other organs, less delicate and less light, require more of the latter than of the former.[1] The *spirituous* blood, more subtile, is contained in the thick-walled arteries, the *venous* and denser blood runs in the veins, the tunics of which are thin.

All the organs which require more venous than spirituous blood (that is to say, all the organs except the lungs) receive the spirituous blood through the arteries, the dense walls of which allow only the most subtile portion, the *spirit*,[2] to escape, and they receive the venous blood by the veins which allow the liquid to escape through their thin walls.[3]

(1) ......Pulmonis corpus leve est, ac rarum, et velut ex spumâ quâdam sanguineâ concretâ conflatum, ob eamque causam puro sanguine, et vaporoso, ac tenui indiguit, non autem, quomodo jecur, limoso et crasso. (*De usu partium*, p. 151.)

(2) ......Nihil nisi tenuissimum sinit elabi. (*Ibid*, p. 151.

(3) ......Quod ergo satius fuit in toto animalis corpore sanguinem quidem tenui ac rarâ, spiritum vero crassâ ac densâ concludi tunicâ, longâ egere ratione non arbitror: satis enim puto esse substantiæ utriusque rationem ac differentiam obiter indicare; quod silicet sanguis quidem crassus est, gravis, agræque mobilis, spiritus vero tenuis, et levis, et citus; quodque periculum erat ne hic expiraret repente, atque, evolaret ab animali, nisi crassis, et densis, atque undique constrictis asservatus fuisset tunicis, atque coercitus: contra vero in sanguine, nisi tenuis et rara fuisset quem ipsum continet tunica, non facile circumfusis partibus distribueretur. (*Ibid.*)

On the contrary, the lungs, which need much more of the spirituous blood than of the venous, receive this kind of blood by a vein, (or, to speak like Galen, by an artery which has the coats of a vein; the *venous artery,*) and the venous blood by an artery (or, again to follow Galen, by a vein which has the coats of an artery, the *arterial vein.*)

This has reference to the adult; let us pass to the fœtus.

It is the spirituous blood which gives to the lungs of the adult that fine, delicate and reticulated structure, which may be said to be formed of the foam of the blood: *velut ex quâdam sanguineâ concretâ spumâ conflatum.*

But the lungs have no need of this peculiar[1] tissue until after birth. After birth they move—before birth they are motionless. They then need only the same structure and the same blood as the other organs; then like the other organs they are thick, gross and red, and then by a singular arrangement they receive like them, more *venous* than *spirituous blood.*[2] How can such a change take place? It is made by means of these two

(1) ......Constructionem ipsius fecerit *eximiam* præter reliquas omnes animalis partes. (*De usu partium,* p. 151.)

(2) At cur pulmo in iis, qui adhuc utero geruntur, est ruber, non autem, ut in perfectis animalibis, subalbus? quia tunc nutritur (quemadmodum reliqua viscera) per vasa

communications—two openings in the heart of the fœtus which do not exist in the heart of the adult—the *ductus arteriosus* and the *foramen ovale.*

These two openings change everything, as far as the lungs are concerned, in the course of the blood in the fœtus. In the adult the *venous artery* carries to the lungs the *spirituous blood* which it has received from the left ventricle (the ventricle in which the *spirits* are formed) in the fœtus the *venous artery* carries to the lungs the *venous blood* which it receives directly from the vena cava, by the *foramen ovale.*[1] In the adult the *arterial vein* carries to the lung the venous blood which it has received from the vena cava, in the fœtus the *arterial vein* carries to the lungs the spirituous blood which it has received from the aorta by the *ductus arteriosus.*

unicam tunicam, et eam tenuem habentia; ad ea nam ex venâ cavâ sanguis pervenit, quo tempore fœtus utero gestatur: in natis vero occæcatur quidem vasorum perforatio,...... quin etiam pulmo tunc motu perpetuo agitatur,... æquum est igitur hic quoque naturam admirari, quæ cum viscus augeri duntaxat oporteret, sanguinem purum ei suppeditabat; cum verò ad motum fuit translatum, carnem levem......fecit...... ob eam igitur causam in fœtibus vena cava in arteriam venosam est pertusa. (*De usu partium*, p. 156.)

(1) Probavimus......... in fœtibus necessarium esse, cum arteria venosa sanguinem a venâ cavâ occipiat, trahi ex eâ non minimum. (*Ibid*, p. 156.)

Between the fœtus and the adult there is then the widest difference.

In the adult the lung receives much *spirituous* blood and little *venous*, in the fœtus much *venous* and little *spirituous*; in the adult the spirituous blood reaches the lungs through the *venous artery*, in the fœtus by the *arterial vein;* in the adult the venous blood arrives by the *arterial vein*, in the fœtus by the *venous artery;* thus the effect of the ductus arteriosus and foramen ovale is to invert the course of the blood and directly changes the functions of the two vessels, giving to the venous artery the functions of the arterial vein and *vice versa.*

Harvey.

Galen supposed that the blood passed through the *foramen ovale*, its course being from the right auricle to the left and from the left auricle through the pulmonary vein into the lungs. But this is not the case; the blood flows through the *foramen ovale* in order to pass from the right auricle into the left, and from the left auricle into the left ventricle, from thence into the aorta, and so on to all parts of the body, escaping the passage through the lungs. He also supposed that the blood passed through the *ductus arteriosus* from the aorta into the pulmonary artery and thence into the lungs. Neither is this the truth.

It goes from the pulmonary artery by the ductus arteriosus into the aorta, and from thence to all parts of the body, again escaping a passage through the lungs. In a word, the *foramen ovale* and the *ductus arteriosus* are not designed to afford a different route by which the blood may reach the lungs in the fœtus from the adult as Galen believed, but their object is to prevent it going to the lungs at all.[1]

In the adult there are two circulations the *pulmonary* and the *general:* in the fœtus there is but one, the *general.* Everything in the adult is arranged in harmony with the existence of two circulations, for neither the two sides of the heart, nor the two great arteries communicate with each other; in the fœtus all is disposed so that there may be but one circulation, for the two sides of the heart, (*i. e.*, the two auricles) open into each other by the *foramen ovale*, and the two great arteries are connected by the *ductus arteriosus.*

In the adult, the two sides of the heart being completely separated, the blood can not pass from one to the other without making the circuit through the lungs; there is, therefore, in the adult a pulmonary circulation; in the fœtus, where the two sides of the heart communicate, the blood passes

(1) Or, at least, that only the least possible quantity may reach them; in truth only that can go there which escapes the *foramen ovale* and the *ductus arteriosus.*

directly from one side to the other through the foramen ovale,[1] and there is, therefore, no pulmonary circulation.

The great point in the adult is, that the blood goes to the lungs because it is by the lungs that the adult respires; the great point in the fœtus is that respiration is not performed by the lungs and, therefore, the blood does not go to them. The fœtus respires by means of another organ.[2]

The lungs of the fœtus do not respire—they do not dilate. They can not then receive the blood of the general circulation; and they do not receive it, through the agency of the foramen ovale and ductus arteriosus, as was so well seen by Harvey, the most ingenious man of the whole world in drawing from the *structure* of parts inferences as to their *uses*.[3]

(1) And also directly from the *pulmonary artery* to the *aorta* by the ductus arteriosus.

(2) By the *placenta* in viviparous animals; by the vessels of the *allantois* in oviparous.

(3) Ex quibus intelligitur in embryone humano,...... id ipsum accidere, ut cor suo motu, per patentissimas vias sanguinem de venâ cavâ in arteriam magnam apertissime traducat, per utriusque ventriculi ductum. Dexter si quidem sanguinem ab auriculâ recipiens, inde per venam arteriosam, et propaginem suam (canalem arteriosum dictam) in magnam arteriam propellit. Sinister similiter eodem tempore, mediante auriculæ motu, recipit sanguinem (in illam sinistram auriculam deductum scilicet per foramen ovale è venâ cavâ),

Duverney and Méry.

Harvey's work appeared in 1628. In 1699, more than half a century later, and when all the teachings of that great man, as well upon the fœtal as upon the adult circulation, had been adopted, and for some time adopted, there arose all at once a very lively discussion in our Academy touching the route which the blood follows in the heart of the fœtus.

In this celebrated discussion between two anatomists of profound ability, Méry and Duverney, Méry was constantly wrong and Duverney as constantly right. Méry was a man of great talent but not of as good judgment as Duverney. The saying of Méry has been preserved for us by Fontenelle: "We anatomists are like the coachmen of Paris who know all the streets, even the smallest and least frequented, but who know nothing of what is taking place in the houses."

Méry admitted that the blood which passes through the *ductus arteriosus* goes from the pulmonary artery to the aorta, and consequently escapes the lungs, as Harvey taught. The difficul-

et tensione suâ, et constrictione per radicem aortæ in magnam itidem arteriam simul impellit....Ita in embryonibus, dum pulmones otiantur, et nullam actionem aut motum habent, quasi nulli forent, natura duobus ventriculis cordis quasi uno utitur, ad sanguinem transmittendum......(Gul. Harvei *Exercit. anat. de motu cordis*, etc., cap. vi.)

ty was only in regard to the *foramen ovale.* According to Harvey the blood which passes through this opening, flows from the right auricle to the left. Méry held to the contrary, that it passed from the left auricle into the right.

Duverney sustained the opinion of Harvey.

The foramen ovale is at first completely open. Soon a delicate membrane commences to form at its edges, which increases and extends itself by degrees, until finally it closes the opening entirely. Now this membrane is disposed in such a manner as to allow the blood to pass from the right into the left auricle, and to resist on the contrary, its motion in the opposite direction.

This Harvey had already observed before Duverney,[1] and Galen before Harvey.[2]

"The mechanism of the valve of the foramen

(1) Insuper in illo foramine ovali è regione, quæ arteriam venosam respicit, operculi instar membrana tenuis et dura est, foramine major, quæ postea in adultis, operiens hoc foramen, et coalescens undique, istud omnino obstruit, et prope obliterat. Hæc, inquam, membrana sic constituta est ut, dum laxe in se concidit,...... sanguini à cavâ affluenti cedat quidem, at ne rursus in cavam refluat, impediat: ut liceat existimare in embryone sanguinem continuò debere per hoc foramen transire de venâ cavâ in arteriam venosam, inde in auriculum sinistram cordis, et postquam ingressum fuerit, remeare nunquam posse. (Gul. Harvei *Exercit, anat. de motu cordis,* etc., p. 44.)

(2) See note 2 page 46.

ovale in the fœtus," says Duverney, "is always such as to allow a free passage of the blood from the vena cava into the left auricle of the heart, and to prevent its return."

He says in another place, "the valve of the foramen ovale of the fœtus, allows the blood to pass easily from the vena cava on into the vein of the lungs, but it entirely prevents its return."

Farther, "the ductus arteriosus of the fœtus serves to relieve the lungs by conducting the greater part of the blood of the pulmonary artery into the aorta."

Finally, he says, "in regard to the human fœtus, which does not respire so long as it is in the body of the mother, if the blood furnished by the two venæ cavæ circulated through the lungs, it would be exposed to fatal accidents; it was necessary then for nature to provide special routes for the relief of the lungs, and she has made these by means of the foramen ovale and the ductus arteriosus."[1]

All these ideas are clear and correct; but Duverney did not stop here. From this study so well pursued, from this clear conception of the circulation of the blood in the fœtus, he extended his investigations to subjects the most important and the most novel—the action of the air in respira-

(1) Mem. de l'Acad. des Sciences, 1699.

tion, and the part which respiration plays in the different classes of animals.

Harvey had already felt the intimate connection between the circulation and the respiration. The question should now be, he says, to know why the blood passes through the lungs in the adult, and why it does not pass through them in the fœtus; why this is necessary in man and in animals which like him are *warm-blooded*, and why it is not necessary, (or at least not so completely) in those that are *cold-blooded*, such as the turtle and the frog. May it be that in man and other warm-blooded animals the blood is so hot that it would *ignite*, *inflame*, perhaps, if it did not go to the lungs to mix with air and be cooled ?[1]

We see then that Harvey did not yet suspect any other use for respiration than that of cooling the blood; and undoubtedly the discoveries of modern chemistry were necessary in order to

(1) Restat ut illud perquiramus...... Aut cur melius sit in adolescentibus, sanguinis transitu naturam omnino occlusisse vias patentes illas, quibus antè in embryone et fœtu usa fuerat...... Cur in majoribus et perfectioribus animalibus, iisque adultis, natura sanguinem transcolari per pulmonum parenchyma potius velit quam ut in cæteris animalibus... Sive hoc sit quod majora et perfectiora animalia sint calidiora, et cum sint adulta, eorum calor magis (ut ita dicam) igniatur et ut suffocetur sit proclivis, et ideo tranare et trajici per pulmones, ut inspirato aere contemperetur, et ab ebullitione et suffocatione vindicetur...... (G. Harvey *Opera*, p. 47.)

pass with certainty from this idea to the opposite one of respiration being the source of the *heat* of the blood. Meanwhile a close and attentive observation of the facts of comparative anatomy would also conduct to this opposite and novel view; by this means Duverney arrived at it.

"When we consider," says Duverney, "that the blood of the pulmonary vein is of a brighter tint than that of the pulmonary artery, we easily conclude that it is charged with some particles of air."[1]

"It is in the lungs," he adds, "that the air communicates to the blood those particles so active and penetrating, upon which its heat depends; it is by this mixture that it is rendered fit for nourishment. We need not be astonished that it is necessary for man, a being of so many different, violent and long continued sensations and movements, for all the blood to circulate through the lungs, but it is sufficient for the turtle and other similar animals, such as the frog and the salamander, which pass all the winter in a state of repose, and which have only sluggish movements, for a third part of the blood to pass through the lungs."[2]

Finally, he wrote this sentence: "The principal function of the lungs is to impregnate the blood

(1) *Mém. de l'Acad. des sc.*, 1701, p. 238.
(2) *Ibid*, 1699, p. 248.

with air, and thus to render it capable of carrying everywhere nutriment, life and heat."[1]

It was not possible to approach nearer to the truth.

In these two chapters, I have studied the discovery of the circulation of the blood properly speaking; it remains for me to consider the discovery of the *lacteals* and of the reservoir of the chyle, *receptaculum chyli;* this will occupy the following chapter.

(1) *Mem. de l'Acad. des. sc.*, 1701, p. 240.

III.

ASELLI,—PECQUET,—RUDBECK,—BARTHOLIN.

The lacteals, the receptaculum chyli, and the lymphatics.

I HAVE already said that modern physiology dates from the discovery of the circulation of the blood.

This discovery Harvey made in 1619 and taught it publicly until 1628 when he published it in his book;[1] and about this time a new influence, the divine breath of discovery, animated all minds; Aselli discovered the lacteals in 1622; Pecquet the receptacle of the chyle in 1648; Rudbeck and Thomas Bartholin the lymphatics between 1650 and 1652. Nothing can be more astonishing than this first outburst of modern genius.

The ancients knew nothing of the lacteals, the lymphatic vessels or the reservoir of the chyle.

Galen believed that the chyle was taken up by the veins of the intestines, and carried by these veins to the liver, and that in the liver it was changed into blood. He believed also that it was

(1) "Per novem et amplius annos multis ocularibus demonstrationibus in conspectu vestro confirmatum."—(See his *Dedication*, p. 1.)

in the liver that the change of blood from black to red took place.

The liver was then at once the organ for converting the chyle into blood and changing black blood into red; the liver was the organ of *sanguification.*

The theory of *sanguification*, of the formation of blood by the liver, was Galen's great theory and great error. It was a learned error, (and such are the most tenacious), which commenced with Galen, was victorious over Harvey, and did not submit until attacked by Pecquet. It was an error for whose dissipation all the discoveries I have just mentioned were necessary, that of the lacteals, that of the lymphatics, and that of the receptaculum chyli; and not only these but others, such as the true uses of respiration, the real action of the air upon the blood, and the true use of the heart.

This singular succession of discoveries remains for us to consider.

Galen and the theory of sanguification.

The theory of sanguification was made up of four points, as I have just said: the first, that the chyle was taken up by the veins of the intestines; the second, that these veins carried it to the liver; the third, that in the liver it was changed into blood; and the fourth, that by the same organ black blood was changed into red.

But to these four points two others were joined; the formation of *spirits*, and the maintenance of *animal heat.*

1 and 2. As fast as the chyle is formed in the stomach and intestines, says Galen, the veins take it up and carry it to a central and common place, which is the liver.[1]

Galen very ingeniously compared the veins of the intestines to the roots of a tree; the smaller uniting to larger ones, these to larger still, and so on to the liver where all were united into one called the *vena porta*,[2] because it is the *gate* of the liver, the gate through which everything passes that arrives at the liver.[3]

(1) "Prius elaboratum in ventriculo alimentum venæ ipsæ deferunt ad aliquem concoctionis locum communem totius animalis, quem hepar nominamus."—(*De usu partium*, lib. iv., p. 135.)

(2) "Colligens vero natura, ut in arboribus, exiguas illas radices in crassiores, ita in animalibus vasa minora in majora, et ea rursus in alia majora, idque semper agens usque ad hepar, in unam omnia venam coegit, quæ ad portas sita est."—(*Ibid.*, p. 141.) *Quæ ad porta sita est*; literally, *which is situated at the gate of the liver.* But this place is the gate of the liver only because it receives the *vena porta*, and all which it conveys or brings. "The *vena porta*, thus named by the ancients, because they believed that it carried the chyle to the liver to be converted into blood."—(*Dionis: Anatomie de l'homme suivant la circulation*, etc., 5th ed., p. 205.)

(3) "Quemadmodum in urbes nihil nisi per portas invehi potest: ita nihil potest in jecur deferri, nisi prius in hunc feratur locum.—(*De constitut. art. med.*, p. 41.)

3. Having reached the liver the chyle ferments there, is concocted, divests itself of its impurities and changes into blood, in the same manner as the *must* in the vats ferments, clears itself of foul matters and changes into wine:[1] "and in the same way," says Descartes, "that the juice of the black grape, which is white, turns into claret wine when the husks remain in the vats with it."

And remark, that the liver has everything necessary for purification, for it has the gall-bladder, the spleen and the kidneys;[2] the gall-bladder which attracts and receives the lightest of the impurities, the spleen which removes the thickest, and the kidneys the more aqueous parts.[3]

4. The chyle which the liver receives is not yet blood, but only an obscure form of blood;[4] in the

(1) "Porro, juxtà exempli similitudinem, intellige mihi distributum à ventriculo ad hepar chylum, à visceris caliditate, velut vinum ipsum in dolio musteum, fervere, concoqui, et alterari in sanguinis boni generationem."—(*De usu partium*, lib. iv., p. 136.

(2) "......... Excrementorum expurgatoria instrumenta: renes, lienem, bilisque receptricem vesicam."—(*De Hipp. et Plat. decret.*, lib. vi.)

(3) "Vesicam, quæ leve et flavum superfluum receptura erat, natura imposuit hepati; splenem verò qui crassum et limosum ...., renes tenue hoc et acquosum excrementum." —(*De usu partium*, lib. iii., p. 136.

(4) "Ipsum autem hepar, postquam id nutrimentum acceperit, ... obscuramque speciem sanguinis referens, inducit

liver the chyle undergoes its last change and purification, and becomes perfect blood, taking on the red color.[1]

The constant merit of Galen was to have coherent and consistent ideas; his constant fault was that he did not verify his ideas by observation. Here, for example, the most simple experiment would have shown him how greatly he was deceived. He had only to expose the liver in a living animal and he would have seen the blood enter it black and leave it of the same color. This single experiment would have led him to suspect his whole theory.

5. *The formation of spirits.* Galen enumerated three kinds of spirits—the *natural*, the *vital*, and the *animal*.

He was not as positive of the existence of the *natural* as of the other two; but in case they did exist he located them in the liver;[2] the *vital* he

ei postremum ornamentum ad sanguinis exacti generationem." —(*De usu partium*, p. 135.)

(1) Et ab innatâ caliditate concretionem exactam est adeptus, ruber jam et purus sursum ad gibbas partes hepatis ascendit."—(*Ibid.*, p. 136.) "Sanguinis rubri prima in jecore generatio est."—(*De Hipp. et Plat. decret.*, lib. vi., p. 266.)

(2) "Quod si naturalis quoque aliquis spiritus est, utique is quoque in jecore et venis continebitur."—(*De methodo medendi*, lib. xii., p. 77.

placed in the heart;[1] the *animal* in the brain;[2] and he accounted for the origin of the two kinds of whose existence he was sure, in the following manner, both being formed from the blood.[3]

The vital spirits are the exhalation of the blood.[4] They are formed in the heart, of the vapor of the blood, particularly in the left ventricle,[5] and from these vital spirits, carried in the arteries[6] to the brain[7] and there more completely elaborated, ripened, and perfected, are formed the *animal spirits.*

(1) "Vitalis spiritus et in arteriis et in corde gignitur."—(*De Hipp. et Plat. decret.*, lib. vii., p. 269.)

(2) "Animalis spiritus cerebrum, veluti fontem esse......... demonstravimus."—(*De methodo medendi*, lib. xii., p. 77.)

(3) "Sicut autem vitalis spiritus secundum arterias et cor generatur, ... ità animalis ex vitali amplius elaborato habet generationem."—(*De virtut. corp. disp.*, p. 61.)

(4) "Spiritus exhalatio quædam sanguinis benigni."—(*De usu partium* lib. vi., p. 155.)

(5) "Copiosior, in sinistro, spiritus substantia."—(*Ibid.*, lib. vi., p. 154.)

(6) "Ab arteriis quibus in ipsum cerebrum acclivis est positio, effluit semper spiritus, belle in retiformi plexu confectus, ... proinde in his moratus diutissime, conficitur; confectus autem statim cerebri ventriculis incidit."—(*Ibid.*, lib. ix., p. 172.)

(7) "Consentaneum igitur rationi est spiritum hunc in cerebri ventriculis oriri."—(*De Hip. et Plat. decret.*, lib. vii., p. 269.)

"Similarly," says Jean Canappe in his quaint language, "hath nature, making from the vital spirits the animal, fashioned and fabricated close to the brain the *rete mirabile*, like unto a labyrinth in which they are elaborated. And afterward they are sent and transmitted to the anterior ventricles where they are still better prepared and rectified: and thence they pass by the common conduit to the posterior ventricle where they receive perfect elaboration."[1]

The *animal* or *cerebral spirit*, the spirit born of the brain, is the most noble and most perfect part of man; it is the substance of the soul itself, or at least its immediate instrument:[2] reason, which is the distinguishing mark of man is seated in the brain,[3] and hence, says Galen, originated the ingenious fable of the birth of Minerva from the brain of Jupiter, which implies that the brain is the source of all the productions of human genius, of all our arts and all our sciences.[4]

(1) *L'anatomie du corps humain*, etc., p. 83.

(2) "Oportet .... hunc ipsum spiritum, aut ipsam animæ substantiam esse, aut primum ipsius instrumentum."—(*De utilitate respirationis*, p. 225.)

(3) "At ratio, quæ revera homo est, sedem in cerebro habens ...." (*De usu partium*, lib. iv., p. 139.)

(4) "Fabula quæ ex Jovis capite Minervam, hoc est prudentiam, natam esse ait ...." (*De Hipp. et Plat. decret.*, lib. iii., p. 247.)

6. *Animal heat.* According to Galen, animal heat is a primitive force, natural and innate.[1] The heart is the source of this heat.[2] From the heart arises the heat of the blood, and from the blood that of the body.[3] Of all parts of the body the heart is the warmest;[4] and of the heart itself the warmest part is the left ventricle;[5] and therefore this ventricle is the place in which the *spirits* are formed, the place where the *venous* blood is changed into *spirituous.*

But for this heat, natural and innate, to be durable an *aliment* was necessary, and in order that it should not become excessive, a *moderator.* The aliment is the blood;[6] the blood, says Galen, is *the*

(1) "Calorem autem non acquisitum .... verum ipsum primum, primogenitum et insitum."—(*De trem., palp., convuls*, etc., p. 54.)

(2) "Cor caloris nativi, quo animal regitur, quasi fons quidem, ac focus est."—(*De usu partium*, lib. vi., p. 150.)

(3) "Sanguis verò ipse à corde suum accipit calorem."—(*De temperamentis*, lib. i., p. 15.) "Et ità calor continuè effluit à corde ad arterias, et per arterias ad totum corpus."—(*De utilit. respirat.*, p. 69, t. vii.)

(4) "Id viscus (cor) tum omnium animalis partium maximè sanguineum, tum vero calidissimum est."—(*De temperamentis*, p. 15.)

(5) "Hunc maximè sinum ad summum pervenire caloris ...." (*De inæquali intemperie*, p. 44.)

(6) "Non solum nutrimentum animantis partibus ex sanguine est, sed calor quoque naturalis perseverantiam ex sanguine obtinet."—(*De curandi ratione per sang. mission.*, p. 16.)

wood of the fire which burns in the heart;[1] and the lungs[2] act as moderator and draw unceasingly by respiration new air into the body and with this air *cool* and temper the heart continually.[3]

The theory of sanguification is now before us.

Nothing could be more complete, for it commenced with the formation of the chyle and only finished with the formation of the *animal spirits*, the instrument of the soul.

And nothing could be better connected, for each step of the process proceeded naturally from the one preceding; the aliment taken into the body was converted into chyle by the stomach and intestines; blood was formed from this chyle in the liver; the vital spirits were exhalations from the blood in the heart, and the animal spirits were elaborated from the vital in the brain. Finally, the blood acquired its temperature from the heart; and the heart found in the blood the *aliment* for its *innate* heat.

But nothing could be more false.

Of all these ideas, these views so well arranged, of this theory so well constructed, and of all this

(1) "Quemadmodum ex lignis comburi idóneis qui in foco est ignis ...." (*De curandi ratione per sang. mission.*, p. 16.)

(2) "Respirationem ingeniti caloris moderationem servare ...." (*De morb. vulg.*, com. v., p. 190.)

(3) "Refrigerat ipsum (cor) inspiratio quidem, frigidam qualitatem ei affundens."—(*De usu partium*, lib. vi., p. 148.)

ingenious labor of the human mind, nothing was true and nothing remains. Galen was not right upon a single point. He said that the chyle is taken up by the veins, which is not so; that it goes to the liver, which is not so; that in the liver the blood changes from black to red, and that is not so, while his *spirits* are but a word, and his *innate heat* only a dream.

Voltaire said that a Frenchman who in his time went from Paris to London *found things much changed;* he left the world full, he found it empty; he left a philosophy which explained everything by *impulse* and found one that accounted for all by *attraction*, etc.

We must admit that if Galen could revisit us and examine physiology now he would also *find things much changed!* He believed that the chyle was carried by veins, and he would be told that there are special vessels for its transmission very distinct from the veins; he thought the chyle went to the liver, he would learn now that it goes to the heart; he believed that the change in the blood from black to red took place in the liver, he would see now that it takes place in the lungs; he was very sure of at least two kinds of spirits, the *vital* and the *animal*, and now he would be told that these spirits are chimeras; finally, he believed that animal heat was an innate primitive property, seated in the heart, and continually tempered, *cooled*, by the lungs, now he would learn that the heart has no such property, that it is but a muscle, and that the lungs, instead of being an organ for *cooling* the heat of the heart are even the source of the heat of that and of all other organs, and that no such thing as innate heat exists in the body.

Aselli and the lacteals.

The ancients knew of only three kinds of vessels, veins, arteries, and nerves (which they took for vessels).[1] The veins conducted the *blood properly speaking*, the arteries the *spirituous blood*, and the nerves the *animal spirits*.[2]

Such was the condition of things. Harvey had not yet published his book, for it was in 1622, when all at once the report spread that an anatomist of Cremona, a professor of Pavia, had just discovered

(1) Notwithstanding Galen's teachings; he knew well enough that the nerves are not hollow: "Nervi qui à cerebro ac spinali medullâ oriuntur nullam habent perspicuam cavitatem."—(*De usu partium*, lib. xv., p. 210.) He was only deceived in regard to the optic nerves: "Solis his nervis, antequam in oculos inserantur, apertè intùs sensibilis quidem meatus adest."—(*De nervorum dissectione*, p. 53.)

(2) "Sic venæ sanguinem distribuunt, arteriæ sanguinem cum spiritu vitali permixtum, nervi animalem spiritum."—(Aselli: *De lactibus, sive lacteis venis, quarto vasorum mesaraïcorum genere dissertatio*, 1627, p. 51.)

a fourth order of vessels[1]—white vessels,—vessels distinct from arteries, veins and nerves and which convey the chyle.

Imagine, if it is possible in our day, the effect produced by such news. The whole world of science was moved by it. The ancients had not then seen all—had not described everything; one now could go farther than Galen and than Aristotle; the wisdom of antiquity was no longer the boundary of human knowledge, and the spirit of modern discovery had commenced its career.

Aselli has told us himself, and in a most simple manner, how the great discovery—the first, strictly speaking, of modern discoveries—(for, I repeat, Harvey's book had not yet appeared,) was made, and accidentally made.[2]

He had just demonstrated upon a living dog, and less for himself than for the benefit of some friends, the *recurrent nerves*. From the recurrent nerves he was requested to pass to the movements of the diaphragm. He opened the abdomen and

(1) "Præter tria illa vasorum genera mesenterium peragrantium (the *veins*, the *arteries* and the *nerves*,) reliquum aliud est genus, quartum, novum, ac ignotum hactenus."—(*De lactibus*, etc., p. 18.)

(2) "A me primo, quod relegatâ omni ambitione dixerim, abhinc fere triennium, hoc est anno adeò 1622, casu magis, ut verum fatear, quam consilio, aut datâ in id peculiari operâ, observatum,"—(*Ibid*, etc., p. 18.)

immediately exposed a most beautiful network of white vessels.[1]

What were these vessels? Could they be vessels for the chyle? That was the inspiration of genius! Aselli pricked one of them; he saw a white liquid exude, and in a transport of joy which can well be conceived, he cried with Archimedes—"*Eureka!*"[2]

But the animal died and all disappeared. Aselli opened another dog; no white vessels were to be seen! Could he have been mistaken? Happily he remembered that the first dog had eaten heartily

(1) "Canem, ad diem julii 23 ejusdem anni, benè habitum, benèque pastum, incidendum vivum sumpseram, amicorum quorumdam rogatu, quibus recurrentes nervos videre fortè placuerat. Eâ nervorum demonstratione perfunctus quum essem, visum est eodem in cane, eâdem operâ, diaphragmatis quoque motum observare. Hoc dum conor, et eam in rem abdomen aperio, intestinaque cum ventriculo collecta in unum deorsum manu impello, plurimos repente, eosque tenuissimos, candidissimosque, ceu funiculos, per omne mesenterium et per intestina, infinitis propemodum propaginibus dispersos, conspicio."—(*De lactibus*, etc., p. 19.)

(2) "Rei novitate perculsus, hæsi aliquandiù tacitus, cum menti variæ occurrerent quæ inter anatomicos versantur, de venis mesaraïcis, et eorum officio controversiæ; .... ut me collegi experiendi causâ, adacto acutissimo scalpello, unum ex illis et majorem funiculum pertundo. Vix benè ferieram, et confestim liquorem album, lactis aut cremoris instar, prosilire video. Quo viso, cum tenere lætitiam non possem, conversus ad eos qui aderant: *Eureka*, inquam, cum Archimede........." (*Ibid.*, p. 19.)

just before the experiment, while the second one was fasting. He took another and fed him well; some hours afterward he opened its abdomen and the white vessels were evident, as in the first one.[1]

The existence of these white vessels, of the vessels of the chyle, was no longer doubtful. Aselli named them *lacteals,* because they contain a white liquid similar to milk.[2] This liquid is the *chyle,* and these lacteal vessels alone convey the chyle;[3] the veins have nothing to do with it.

(1) "Verum eo diu frui non licuit. Exspiravit mox inter hæc canis, et unà (dictu miram) omnis illa tot vasorum series congeriesque defecta candore suo, defecta succo, inter manus ipsas nostras ac penè inter oculos ità evanuit, vix ut vestigia sui relinqueret .... Conquisitus ergò canis alius in diem posterum, et nullâ interpositâ morâ die eodem apertus. Porrò minimè, ut spes, ità successus fuit. Nullum prorsus, vel minimum album vasculum in conspectum sese dabat. Et jam abjici anomo cœperam .... Verum in memoriam revocans, siccum et impastum fuisse canem, quem secandum arripueram, suspicatusque, quod res erat, ne intestinorum inanitas causa fuisset vasorum obliterationis, etiam tertiò rem periclitari volui, alio rursus in id comparato cane. Is sectus ad diem 26, horâ circiter sextâ postquam cibus illi adhibitus affatim fuerat, ... nihil fefellit expectatio. Omnia quæ primus luculenter et adamussim exhibuit .... Confirmatus gemino hoc experimento, et nihil amplius de re ipsâ ambigens, totum me dedi ad perquirendam eam."—(*De lactibus*, p. 19.)

(2) "Ego vasa hæc, aut lacteas, sive albas venas, aut lactes etiam appellare soleo."—(p. 23.) "Non lac ipsum magis simile lacti est quam liquor qui in illis cernitur."—(p. 25.)

(3) "Chylus per eas labitur; verissime idem ex intestinis ab iis lacitur, hoc est sorbetur exhauriturque."—(p. 25.)

Pecquet and the reservoir of the chyle.

The lacteals then convey the chyle; but where do they carry it? Aselli believed it was to the liver. "The use of our *veins*," says he, "is without any doubt to carry the chyle, and also without any doubt to carry it to the liver."[1]

The chyle, therefore, still went to the liver, and Galen's principal error (the principal because all the others depended upon it, the liver being supposed the organ of *sanguification* only because the chyle was carried to it,) existed still. But it could not maintain its ground much longer.

In 1648,[2] a young man of Dieppe, who had studied medicine at Montpelier, Jean Pecquet, tired of *cold and dumb*[3] facts derived from the dead organs of the subject, and desiring more correct knowledge,[4] asked it of the living.

He commenced a series of experiments and researches upon living animals. He opened the

(1) "Actio propria venarum nostrarum, alisque omni dubitatione, chyli distributio ad jecur."—(*De lactibus*, p. 51.)

(2) "......... Assiduum ferme trium annorum laborem coarctavi."—(*Experimenta nova anatomica, quibus ignotum hactenus chyli receptaculum, et ab eo per thoracem in ramos usque subclavios vasa lactea deteguntur*, 1651, p. 17.)

(3) "Post acquisitam ante annos aliquot, ex cadaverum sectione, mutam alioqui frigidamque sapientiam."—(p. 4.)

(4) "Placuit ex vigenti vivorum animantium harmoniâ verum scientiam experimere."—(p. 4.)

thorax of a dog; in taking out the heart he observed in the midst of the flowing blood a white liquid which he at first took for pus.[1] A little study convinced him that this white and milky liquid was the same as that contained in the lacteals—was the *chyle*[2]; and farther observation showed that it was contained in the canal which carries it to the subclavian veins and that by these veins it is poured into the heart;[3] another step was to learn that this canal commences by a sort of *reservoir* or pocket,[4] and another that *all the lac-*

(1) "Cor, rescissis quibus reliquo adhæret corpori vasculorum retinaculis, avello; tum exhaustâ quæ statim restagnaverat copiâ cruoris, albicantem subinde lactei liquoris nec certe parum fluidi scaturiginem ...., miror effluere,......... (p. 4) sic ut dilitescentis intrà thoracem fortè saniem abcessus, ex cruenti puris imagine, suspicarer."—(*Experimenta nova anatomica*, etc., p. 5.)

(2) "......... Candidus apprimè liquor, et effuso per mesenterium chylo simillimus; sic ut inter utrumque collatos invicem et nitor et odor et sapor et consistentia nullum inesse discrimen ostenderint."—(p. 5.)

(3) "......... Unicus, crassiorque canalis, à *receptaculo* chylum ad quartam dorsi vertebram devolvit, indeque bifidus per subclaviorum (ut in cane notavimus) ostiola foraminum eumdem in cavum exonerat."—(p. 17.)

(4) "......... Laceratâ forte sinistrorsum ad duodecimam circiter dorsi vertebram ampullâ, cujus est apprimè tenuis membranula, restagnantem demiratus lactis effusi copiam, suspicor non exiguum illic ejusdem liquoris occludi *receptaculum*."—(p. 11.)

teals empty into this reservoir which is thus a common receptacle;[1] and lastly he learned that none of these vessels, absolutely none, go to the liver.[2]

The chyle does not then go to the liver; and since it does not go to that organ can not there be changed into blood; the liver, therefore, is not the organ of *sanguification;*[3] and the theory of Galen, a theory which had lived through fifteen centuries, was finally destroyed.

Rudbeck and the lymphatic vessels; particularly those of the Liver.

But this was not all. One discovery was the cause of another. The discovery of the *lacteals* occasioned that of the *receptaculum chyli*, and this caused the discovery of the lymphatics.

In 1650, and this time again a young man, Olaüs Rudbeck, afterward one of the most learned men of Sweden, sought for the *common trunk* of the

(1) "Sic tandem patuit reconditi chyli penus, et tantis laborimus quæsitum *receptaculum*" .... (*Experimenta nova anatomica*, etc., p. 14.) "Lancinata illico *receptaculi* tunica chylum effudit; et secutus per ejusdem vulneris rimam .... dubium omne revulsit scaturienti evidentia."—(p. 15.)

(2) "Nullus ad jecur porrigi inventus est."—(p. 13.)

(3) "Hactenus e mesenterio chylum in hepatis parenchyma opinio protrusit, non veritas, et sanguineo artificii tribuit immeritam .... visceri prærogativam."—(p. 13.)

lacteal vessels and found it.[1] He did not know that Pecquet had just discovered it. In seeking for this chyle-duct Rudbeck remarked upon the liver certain transparent watery vessels, which he recognized immediately as new and peculiar—as vessels distinct from the lacteals.[2] These vessels were *lymphatics*.

Rudbeck named them *hepatico-aqueous* vessels; hepatic because they came from the liver, and aqueous on account of the transparent fluid which filled them.[3]

He saw their origin, their valves,[4] their termina-

(1) *Nova exercitatio anatomica, exhibens ductus hepaticos aquosos et vasa glandularum serosa* (in Mangeti *Bibliothicâ anatomica.* Genevæ, 1699, t. ii., p. 729.)

(2) "Dum anno 1650 et 1651, in venarum lactearum originem et insertionem inquirendam versabar, injectâque suprà venam portæ cum ductibus cholidocis ligaturâ, non semel apparuere ductus manifestò ab hepate ad ligaturam intumescentes ...." (p. 730.)

(3) "Hæc vasa *ductuum hepaticorum aquosorum* nomine indigitanda duxi: et quidem *ductuum hepaticorum*, quum et humorem ferant ac ducant, et quod illum ab hepate accipiant, indeque suam originem depromant; deinde *aquosorum*, quod tali humore ipsorum cavitas infarta sit."—(p. 730.)

(4) "Figuram .... mirabiliter nodosam, ob contentas valvulas .... (p. 731.) Aselli had seen the valves of the lacteals, "in his illud admiratione dignum, quod pluribus valvulis, sive ostiolis, interstincti sunt." (*De lactibus*, etc., p. 38;) and Pecquet those of the thoracic duct: "Non desunt suæ *lacteis* per thoracem valvulæ."—(*Experim. nov.*, etc., p. 12.)

tion in the receptacle or reservoir of the chyle;[1] and he is the first who observed these points, who discovered; but in regard to the discovery of the lymphatic vessels which are spread everywhere through the system, he is only the second.

Thomas Bartholin and the lymphatics of the entire body.

Rudbeck discovered the lymphatic vessels 1650–51;—Thomas Bartholin discovered them 1651–52;[2] he named them *lymphatic vessels;*[3] he studied them with attention and with admirable perseverance; he sought for them everywhere, and he found them everywhere, in the viscera, in the extremities, etc.,[4] and whatever their origin he saw, with Rudbeck, that they emptied into a common trunk, into the *receptaculum chyli.*[5]

The lymphatics and the lacteals have then a

(1) "In vesiculum chyli .... sese insinuant."—(*Magneti, Bibl. anat.*, t. ii., p. 730.)

(2) "Observavimus quidem sæpe in canibus dissectis, imprimis 15 decemb. 1651, et 9 janu. 1652, ex hepate aquosus ductus prodeuntes .... (*Vasorum lymphaticorum Historia nova, in Opuscula nova*, etc., p. 84.)

(3) "A contenti liquoris conditione, seu limpidâ aquâ et lymphâ, dicenda vasa lymphatica ...." (p. 96.)

(4) "Exortus lymphaticorum vasorum est ab extremis partibus, seu artubus et visceribus ...." (p. 97.)

(5) "Vasa aquosa .... inseruntur in receptaculum chyli ...." (p. 97.)

common trunk and a common receptacle, the reservoir and the duct of the chyle; and by this duct their contents are poured into the subclavian veins and by them carried to the heart.

The heart is, therefore, the common *rendezvous*, the center of the circulatory system. And this system is not composed alone of arteries and veins, as Galen taught, and as Harvey believed, but of arteries, veins, *lacteals* and *lymphatics*. The complete unity of this great system was finally found.

Thomas Bartholin and the obsequies of the liver.

Thomas Bartholin terminates his "*History of the lymphatic vessels*" by a chapter entitled: *Post invento vasa lymphatica hepatis exsequiæ.*

Pecquet having demonstrated that the lacteals do not go to the liver, that the chyle is not taken there, and that the liver, therefore, can not be the organ of *sanguification*, it was time, in the language of Bartholin, to perform the *obsequies* of the liver. But why does not Bartholin speak of their performance before the discovery of the lymphatics? Because the first time he saw the lymphatics of the liver he took them for lacteals going to that organ.[1] The liver then, he says to himself, re-

(1) "Unde quum pellucido liquore splenderent, nec aliud vas cognitum adhuc esset .... tamdiu pro lacteis venditavi .... Exinde dubitare cœpi, visis aquosis ductibus, in artubus, illis similibus ...." (p. 88.)

ceives a part of the chyle-vessels and a portion of the chyle; it must have, therefore, a certain part to play in sanguification; this function must be divided between it and the heart.[1]

But Bartholin soon recognized the true nature of the vessels which had deceived him; they were not *lacteals* but *lymphatics;*[2] instead of going *to* the liver they came *from* it; they led to the heart, and consequently the cause of the liver was forever lost.[3]

Bartholin treated the liver, which he compared to a great hero, *maximus heroïbus,*[4] as all great heroes are treated when their cause is lost, he abandoned it; and in a vein of learned gaiety, after having written its *obsequies,* he composed an epitaph for it, of which the sense is, that the liver, so long famous, by means of an usurped title, is now nothing more than a poor liver reduced to making bile.[5]

(1) "Partitus sum munia cordis et hepatis in opere conficiendi sanguinis, quia ad cor lacteas thoracicas ferri observavi, et ad hepar non nullas .... (p. 108.)

(2) "Vidimus quippe vasa illa propè hepar, sui esse generis, à contento liquore *lymphatica* nobis dicta ...." (p. 109.)

(3) "Noluimus antiquatæ opinioni obstinatiùs inhærere, aut labantes hepatis derelicti partes diutiùs sequi."—(p. 109.)

(4) *Vasorum lymphaticorum,* etc., p. 111.

(5) *Manuel anatomique,* Paris, 1661, p. 688.

Riolan and Harvey.

Harvey had no sooner published his work upon the *circulation of the blood* than twenty anatomists took up the pen against the discovery. Harvey did not reply. The only man to whom Harvey ever did the honor of responding was Riolan. It was because Riolan was the best anatomist of those times. Thomas Bartholin who dedicated to him his "*Histoire des vaisseaux lymphatics,*" calls him the greatest anatomist of France and of the world: *Maximo orbis et urbis Parisiensis anatomico.*

Riolan passed all his life in seeking, in demonstrating, and *discovering* what the ancients had taught, and in opposing the doctrines of the moderns. He rejected the circulation of the blood, the lacteals, the receptaculum chyli and the lymphatics. "Everybody is discovering something new now-a-days," he exclaims;[1] and it was this that grieved him. "Pecquet," he continues, "has done much more; he has commenced to demolish the structure and the composition of the human body by his new and unheard-of doctrines, which completely overturn the science of medicine, ancient and modern, or ours."[2] "*And modern, or ours*" is a curious expression! but, alas! the *modern* belongs to no one; scarcely does it exist before it is past and another *modern* has arrived!

(1) *Manuel anat.*, p. 689. (2) *Ibid.*, p. 689.

Meanwhile, Riolan did not deny the existence of the *lacteals;* but he held still that they went to the liver.[1] Harvey denied up to this time the existence of the lacteals and it is both amusing and singular to find that Riolan reproaches him for it. "Harvey," says he "a very expert anatomist, the author and inventor of the circulation of the blood by the heart and through the lungs, makes but little of these lacteal veins, believing and sustaining the doctrine that the chyle passes by the mesenteric veins, from whence it is drawn by the liver, all of which astonishes me much, since they truly exist and we can plainly see them."[2]

Here then is Harvey, the author of the most beautiful of modern discoveries, reproached by his great adversary Riolan, and reproached for his opposition to modern doctrines!

The illustrious and learned historian of medicine, Sprengel, says on this occasion: "A still greater blot upon the literary character of Harvey is the contempt which he affected for all subsequent discoveries." These words are unjust. Sprengel did not reflect sufficiently upon the extent to which deep reflection exhausts and how much meditation is necessary for a discovery of a certain order.

(1) "For myself, I believe that these lacteal veins are not useless, but that they serve to carry the chyle from the intestines to the liver."—(p. 696.)

(2) *Manuel anatomique*, p. 695.)

Harvey discovered the *circulation of the blood;* he gave us a crowd of facts and views, and an admirable general law on *generation.*[1] After this we should admire him—bless him—and not demand too much of him.

Aristotle and the formation of the blood by the heart.

Galen admitted three principal organs, the liver, the heart, and the brain; from the liver proceeded the veins, from the heart the arteries, and from the brain the nerves. According to Aristotle all these came from the heart: veins, arteries and nerves.[2]

Aristotle believed that the blood was formed in the heart;[3] and this opinion in regard to the formation of the blood by the heart, although for a long time superseded by the contrary opinion of its formation by the liver, remained in science. Servetus makes allusion to it in that immortal passage which I have already cited, where he says: "The yellow color is given to the blood by the lungs and

(1) That every living being proceeds from an egg: *Omne vivum ex ovo.*

(2) "The heart is the source of all the veins."—(*History of animals*, book iii., chap. iv.) "Let us pass to the nerves; they likewise originate in the heart."—(*Ibid.*, chap. v.) Note that Aristotle united under the common name of *veins*, the veins and the arteries.

(3) "The liquid which proceeds from the food flows continally to the heart; it is this liquid which forms blood."—(*Of respiration*, chap. xx.)

not by the heart." Cæsalpinus adopts it completely when he says: "the blood, conducted to the heart by the veins, receives there its last perfection, and this acquired it is carried to all parts of the body."

Thus, so soon as it was proved that the chyle was carried to the heart and not to the liver everybody returned to the opinion of Aristotle, to the belief that the blood was formed by the heart. "This plainly proves," says Pecquet, "the truth of the teachings of the Prince of the Peripateciens, who held the heart to be the origin of the veins, and that it is the organ for the formation of blood."[1] "It is in the heart," says Rudbeck, "that the blood, being brought from all parts of the body is mixed with chyle, elaborated, perfected and colored."[2] Bartholin, as we have just seen, divided the function of sanguification between the liver and the heart.

They escaped one error only to fall into another. Two men however soon combatted this other error.

(1) "......... Sicut evincatur nobili testimonio, quum apposité Peripateticorum princeps, et venarum asserat cor esse principium, et sanguinis officinam."—*Experimenta nova anatomica*, etc., p. 3.)

(2) "Existimo itaque hoc opus naturæ (sanguificationis nempé), hunc in modum fieri. Primò, sanguis à nutritione residuus, et cordi advectus, unà cum chylo, motu ac calore cordis concoquitur, coloratur, attenuatur, ac distribuitur."—(Mangeti, *Bibliotheca anatomica*, t. ii., p. 733.)

Stenon demonstrated the heart to be nothing more than a simple organ of movement—a muscle; and Lower showed that the blood changes its color from black to red in the lungs.

Stenon and the true use of the heart.

Stenon was a man of genius. Deluc called him the *first true geologist*, because he was the first who correctly saw the disposition and structure by *layers*, the regular *stratification* of the surface of the globe; and I call him the *first true anatomist of the brain*, because he was the first who recognized the *fibres* of the brain, that is to say the most important part of the structure of this organ.

"It is certain," says Stenon, "and demonstrable to the eye as well as to the reason, that the heart is a muscle, that it is all a muscle and nothing but a muscle; so that it can be neither the organ of internal heat, nor the seat of the soul; nor does it produce the vital spirits, or the blood, or give origin to any other humor whatever.[1]

(1) "Si certum est, quod certum esse sensuum ope adjuta evincit ratio, in corde nihil desiderari quod musculo datum, nec quod musculo denegatum in corde inveniri, non erit cor amplius sui generis substantia, adeoque nec certæ substantiæ, ut ignis calidi innati, animæ sedes, nec certi humoris, ut sanguinis, generator, nec spirituum quorumdam vitalium productor."—(*De musculis specimen*, p. 523, in Mangeti *Biblioth. anat.*) Stenon's book is dated 1664.

Lower and the coloration of the blood by the lungs; or, rather, by the air.

Lower's book upon the heart is short, full, excellent.[1] His was one of the finest minds ever devoted to physiology. His advances are sure, his views clear, his experiments judicious.

It is evident that the *right* ventricle has the same structure as the left; the same conclusions may therefore be drawn from the one as from the other. On examining now the blood of the *vena cava, i. e.* blood which has not yet traversed the right ventricle, and the blood of the *pulmonary artery* which is just leaving the ventricle, it will be found that they are both just alike; they are both the same blood, the *venous* or *black* blood.[2]

If the trachea of a living animal be tied so that the lung can receive no more air, then the blood of the *carotid artery* will be black like that of the *jugular vein; i. e.* blood which has just come from the left ventricle is the same as that which has not yet arrived there.[3]

(1) It appeared in 1669.

(2) ...... "Quum par sit utriusque ventriculi officium ...... quidni color in dextro pariter immutari debeat? At certò constat sanguinem ex arteriâ pulmonali eductum venoso per omnia similem esse, crassamentum ejus nempe obscuri coloris est .... (*Tractatus de corde*, etc., edition of 1740, p. 184.)

(3) "Quinimò nec à sinistro cordis ventriculo novum hunc ruborem sanguini impertiri certissimo hoc experemínto con-

If, in a dog which has just expired, the yet fluid blood be pushed from the *vena cava* into the lungs, and at the same time air be forced into them, the blood of the *pulmonary veins* immediately becomes red.[1]

Finally, and this is an experiment which is only surpassed in beauty by the finest of Bichat's, if the thorax of a living dog be opened the lungs collapse, receive no more air, and the blood of the *pulmonary veins* is black; if air be forced in, the blood becomes red; if the insufflation be suspended it again becomes black, and again changes to red on the insufflation being recommenced.[2]

fici potest: .... si nimirum aspera arteria in collo nudata discindatur, et immisso subere arctè desuper ligetur, ne quid aeris in pulmones ingrediatur, sanguis ex arteriâ cervicali simul discissâ effluens, ... totus venosus pariter et atri coloris apparebit, non aliter quam si venâ jugulari pertusâ profusus fuisset ...." (p. 184.)

(1) "Postremò, nè quis ultrà vel dubitandi locus supersit, experiri animum subiit in cane strangulato, postquam sensus illum et vita omnis deseruissent, an sanguis adhuc fluidus, è venâ cavâ in dextrum cordis ventriculum et pulmones impulsus, pariter floridus per venam pneumonicam totus rediret; itaque propulso sanguine, atque insufflatis simul .... pulmonibus, exspectationi eventus optimè respondebat, quippe æque purpureus in patinam excipiebatur, ac si ex arteriâ viventis effusus fuisset."—(p. 185.)

(2) "Expertus sum sanguinem, qui totus venosi instar subnigricante colore pulmones intrarat, arteriosum omnino et floridum ex illis rediisse, si enim abscissâ anteriore parte pec-

It is, therefore, in the lungs alone, and by the air alone, that the black blood is changed into red; and of the four principal errors of Galen, not one now remained. All four were destroyed, and the destruction of each is the glory of a different man. Aselli taught us that the chyle is carried by special vessels and not by veins; Pecquet that it goes to the heart and not to the liver; Stenon that the heart is a simple muscle and not the originator of

toris, et folle in asperam arteriam immisso, pulmonibus continenter insufflatis, ... vena pneumonica prope auriculam sinistram pertundatur, sanguis totus purpureus et floridus in admotum vasculum exsiliet; atque quamdiù pulmonibus recens usque aer hoc modo suggeritur sanguis ad plures uncias, imò libras, per totum coccineus erumpet, non aliter quam si ex arteriâ vulneratâ exciperetur ...." (p. 186.) "One of the best methods," says Bichat, "to judge of the change of color of the blood, I believe is the one of which I make use. It consists first in adapting to the divided trachea a stop-cock which may be opened or closed at pleasure; and then in opening an artery, such as the carotid, or the femoral, so as to observe the alterations of color in the blood as it flows out."—(*Recherches physiologiques sur la vie et la mort.—De la mort des organes par celle du poumon*, art. viii. § i.)—"1. Adapt a tube with a stop-cock to the trachea exposed and divided; 2. Open the abdomen so as to expose the intestines, mesentery, etc. 3. Close the stop-cock. At the end of two or three minutes the bright red tint which enlivens the whiteness of the peritoneum and which this membrane derives from the numerous vessels distributed over it, will become dark and dull, and this change may be repeated again and again by opening and closing the stop-cock."—(*Ibid.*, art. vi., § ii.)

heat; Lower demonstrated that it is in the lungs and not in the liver that the elaboration of the blood is completed, and the conversion of the black blood into red takes place.

So much for the four principal errors of the theory of Galen. There remain only two accessory ones—that of the *spirits* and that of *innate heat.* Let us give a rapid glance at the manner of their fall.

The spirits.

We know that of Galen's three kinds of spirit the moderns only adopted one, the *animal spirits.* "The ancients admitted," says Bordeu, "three sorts of spirits; and it is not easy to understand by what fatality the natural and the vital have not been able to maintain themselves and have succumbed, while the animal still subsist."[1] Begging Bordeu's pardon, nothing is easier to understand. It was because Descartes introduced the *animal spirits* into his philosophy, and did not introduce the others. The fortune of the animal spirits in modern times depended entirely upon the philosophy of Descartes. As long as that philosophy existed they remained in being and when it fell they fell with it. I say *when this philosophy*

(1) *Recherches anatomiques sur la position des glandes et sur leur action,* § xxxiv.

fell,—I speak of the exterior of the philosophy, of its forms, of its applications, of its phrases, of the ideas it borrowed from imperfect physiology and physics; for, in regard to the essential, the foundation—its spirit and its method—it can not fall. Far from it; the more we study man, or that which is really man, the reason, the soul, the more we shall appreciate the truth of the philosophy of Descartes, and the we shall feel its greatness and its grandeur.

Innate heat.

Of all the errors of Galen, or, to speak more correctly, of ancient physiology (for this is not alone Galen's error, but that of Aristotle, of Hippocrates, and of all antiquity), that which lasted the longest was the one in regard to *innate heat*. This only gave way before modern chemistry, and then not immediately.

In spite of the miracles of modern chemistry, the decomposition of the air, the separation of the air into respirable and non-respirable portions, showing in the respirable element the cause of the coloration of the blood, and in the decomposition of the air by respiration the source of animal heat, more than one old physiologist resisted still.

Fabre, an ingenious physiologist, but of narrow ideas, (and of which the least worthy is the one which Broussais has borrowed from him, of *irrita-*

tion being the sole cause of all the phenomena of life,) Fabre held that *animal heat* was the simple effect of *irritability* and had for its focus the heart, the most *irritable* organ of the economy.[1]

Barthez, a profound physiologist, but one who saw the origin of physical phenomena in metaphysical causes,[2] maintained animal heat to be an *affection of the vital principle*, a *generative* affection producing the heat,[3] and that the respired air *cooled* the blood.[4]

Fouquet, the great founder of chemical study in France, said of these new theories: "They are the work of youngsters and I am now so old that it is not worth while to make myself acquainted with them." How many men have been able to

(1) "I believe we are able to attribute animal heat to irritability."—(*Essai sur les facultes de l'âme*, 1787, p. 40.) "The heart, on account of the multitude of its fibres, and the force of their contraction, should be regarded as the principal focus from whence emanates that heat which the blood carries to all parts of the body.—(*Ibid.* p. 41.)

(2) Upon this vice of philosophy, see the author's *Histoire des travaux de Buffon*, and his *Histoire de Fontenelle.*

(3) .... "L'affection du principe vital, qui est regeneratrice de la chaleur" .... (*Nouveaux elements de la science de l'homme*, Paris, 1806, t. i., p. 304.)

(4) A la suite des effets que l'air, nouvellement respiré, produit à la surface des vaisseaux aériéns du poumon qu'il rafraichit."—(*Ibid.* p. 303.)

speak thus! And we must add that this Fouquet, so hostile to modern ideas was an ardent supporter of the doctrines of the ancients. Seated in his professional chair he never pronounced the name of Hippocrates without uncovering his head! The erudite of all kinds resemble a little La Bruyere, —they have seen even the Tower of Babel but have not visited Versailles.

IV.

SARPI AND THE VALVES OF THE VEINS.

I have said but a word of Sarpi and that is not enough.

The learned author of a very remarkable analysis of the work of M. Bianchi Giovini upon Sarpi, published in the London and Westminster Review, for April, 1838, has re-opened a question which seemed to have been decided.[1]

First, M. Giovini produces in favor of Sarpi a new document; second, the author to whom I allude, after having placed Harvey's fame in safety (which was his first care,) becomes much less careful in regard to the others, and appears even too compliant when the question is only in regard to Fabricius ab Acquapendente.

I have already said that the discovery of the circulation of the blood does not belong to any single man. This grand discovery was only made little by little and part by part; more than twenty anatomists took part in it.

Harvey demonstrated the circulation of the blood; but he came from Padua, where Fabri-

(1) See on page 33 the opinion of a master in Italian criticism, Tiraboschi.

cius, who had discovered the valves of the veins, was his teacher; in this same university of Padua where were formed the germs of all Harvey's[1] ideas, Realdo Columbus, who discovered the pulmonary circulation, was but a short time before professor; and Padua is not far from Pisa, where Cæsalpinus, by the light of genius caught sight of the pulmonary circulation, and by a brighter flash of the same divine fire saw the general circulation.

In the discovery of the circulation, the point of difficulty was to unite the diverse observations successively made, or so to speak, the different pieces, into one whole; the difficulty was to comprehend the phenomena and the whole of the mechanism united together; and it is because Harvey was the first who clearly and completely comprehended this whole that the glory has remained his.

Sarpi.

There are just two questions relative to Sarpi: the first is to ascertain which of the two, Fabricius or he, discovered the valves of the veins; the

(1) Harvey has left two fundamental works, one on the *circulation* and the other on *generation:* in the first he starts from the discovery of the valves made by Fabricius, and in the second, from the labors of this same Fabricius upon *the formation of the egg and of the fœtus: De formato fœtu et De formatione ovi et pulli.*

second is to learn whether he understood the circulation. According to his partisans he discovered the veins and was acquainted with the circulation; but in my opinion, he neither discovered the one nor knew anything of the other.

Sarpi and the valves of the veins.

It has been said then that Sarpi discovered the valves of the veins. But who says this? It is Father Fulgence, the companion, the friend, the enthusiastic biographer of Father Sarpi.

"Many very learned men and very eminent physicians are living yet," Fulgence tells us, "who know very well that the discovery of the valves does not belong to Fabricius ab Acquapendente, but to the Father S., *ma dal Padre*, who reflecting on the gravity of the blood, came to think that it could not remain *suspended*, as it is in the veins, if it was not supported by some dam or obstacle, and thereupon, he set about making researches and discovered the valves and their use."[1]

(1) Sono ancora viventi molti eruditissimi e eminentissimi medici, tra questi Santorio Santorio e Pietron Asselineo, francese, che sanno che non fu speculatione, ne inventione dell' Acquapendente, ma dal Padre, il quale considerando la gravità del sangue, venne in parere che non potesse stare sospeso nelle vene, senza che vi fosse argine che lo ritenesse, e chiusure, ch' aprendosi et risserrandosi gli dassero il flusso, e l'equilibrio necessario alla vita. E con questo natural

Now then what is this use? According to Fulgence, that is to say according to Sarpi, it is "not alone to prevent the blood by its weight distending the veins and thus causing varices, but by moderating its too rapid course and limiting its quantity to prevent it from destroying the heat of the parts which it should nourish.[1]"

We must at least conclude then, before quitting Fulgence, that Sarpi did not understand the use of the valves. The valves prevent a retrograde flow of blood, but present no obstacle to its rapid advance, and it is scarcely necessary for me to add that the parts are not nourished by the blood of the veins.

After Fulgence comes Gassendi.

"I had no sooner informed him," Gassendi tells us in his life of Peiresc, "that William Harvey, an English physician, had just published a very remarkable book upon the continual passage of the blood from the veins into the arteries and again from the arteries into the veins by imperceptible anastomoses, and that among other arguments to

giuditio si pose à tagliare con isquisitissima osservatione, et ritrovò le valvule, e gl' usi loro......(*Opere del Padre Paolo dell' Ordine dei Servi*, etc., 1687: *Vita dal Padre*, p. 44.)

(1) "Perche non solamente prohibiscono ch'el sangue per la gravita non dilati le vene, a guisa di varice, ma anco á fine che con troppo impeto scorrendo, et in soverchia quantita, non soffochi il calor delle parti, che desso si debbono nutrire." (*Ibid*, p 45.)

confirm this passage, he makes great use of the valves of the veins, of which he himself had learned something from Fabricius ab Acquapendente, than recollecting that Father Sarpi, Servite, was the first inventor, he would have the book and seek out the valves and know all the rest."[1]

Thus then it is Gassendi who reminds Peiresc that Fabricius has spoken to him of the valves of the veins, and he, Peiresc, recollects that it is Sarpi who has discovered them. But who told Peiresc this? Apparently it was not Fabricius. Might it not have been Father Fulgence?

From this "remembrance" of Peiresc let us pass to another point, to some few words written by the rapid and prolix pen of Thomas Bartholin. Bartholin was traveling, and was in Padua at that time; he wrote from that place to Jean Walæus, professor at Leyden; of course there was much to write from Padua. He related then, "that finally he had heard from Vesling the secret of the dis-

(1) Cum simul monuissem Gulielmum Harvæum, medicum Anglum, edidisse præclarum librum de successione sanguinis ex venis in arterias et ex arteriis rursus in venas per imperceptas anastomoses, inter cetera verò argumenta confirmasse illam ex venarum valvulis, de quibus ipse inaudierat aliquid ab Acquapendente, et quarum inventorem primum Sarpium Servitam meminerat, ideò statim voluit et librum habere, et eas valvulas explorare et alia internoscere... (*Viri illustris Nicolai Claudii Fabricii de Peiresc Vita* per Petrum Gassendum ......1641, p. 222.)

covery of the circulation of the blood, a secret which was not to be revealed to anybody; *nulli revellandum;* to-wit: that it was discovered by Father Paul, a Venetian, (from whom also Fabricius had derived the discovery of the valves of the veins) as he had seen by a manuscript of Father Paul's which was at Venice, in the possession of his successor and disciple Father Fulgence."[1] Always Father Fulgence!

Again, why should not this secret be confided to any one? Why even was it a secret at all? It certainly was not a sin to have discovered the circulation of the blood or the valves of the veins. Finally, why reveal it if it ought not to be revealed? Above all, why wait until after Fabricius' death before making this disclosure?[2]

Fabricius did not await the death of Sarpi before saying publicly and plainly that he had discovered the valves. "What first astonishes," says he, "is that these valves have so long escaped anatomists, ancient as well as modern, and so entirely

(1) De circulatione Harvejanâ secretum mihi aperuit Veslingius, nulli revelandum; esse nempe inventum Patris Pauli, veneti (à quo de ostiolis venarum sua habuit Acquapendens,) ut ex ipsius autographo vidit, quod Venetiis servat P. Fulgentius, illus discipulis et successor...... Patavio. 30 oct. 1642. (Thom. Barthol. *Epist. med.* cent. i, epist. xxvi.)

(2) The letter of Thomas Bartholin is dated in 1642, and the death of Fabricius took place in 1619.

escaped them that no mention was made of them, no one had seen them, until the year 1574 when I observed them for the first time with great joy: *summâ cum letitiâ.*" [1]

When Fabricius wrote this Sarpi was twenty-two years old.[2] He lived forty-nine years after Fabricius had made this declaration, yet neither he himself, nor Father Fulgence, nor any other of his friends, ever raised his voice against Fabricius, but all of them as we have just seen, kept their secret close, and advised its farther keeping; they revealed it, however, but unhappily not until after the death of Fabricius.

Add to this, and this is a decisive point, that Fabricius was not only a consummate anatomist and a superior man of science but he was eminently an honest man. Harvey called him a venerable old man; *venerabilis senex.* Says he, "it was the illustrious Jerome Fabricius ab Acquapendente, a most skillful anatomist and venerable old man, who first saw in the veins the membranous valves of sigmoid or semi-lunar shape." [3]

(1) See page 32 ,note 2.

(2) He was born in 1552 and died in 1623.

(3) "Clarissimus Hieronym. Fab. ab Acquapendente, peritissimus anatomicus et venerabilis senex, primus in venis membraneas valvulas delineavit figurâ, sigmoïdes, vel semilunares portiunculas tunicæ interioris venarum, eminentes et tenuissimas... (*Exerc. anat. de motu cordis et sanguinis*, cap. xiii.)

The friends of Sarpi reckon as many as five witnesses for him; first, Fulgence, then Peiresc, next Vesling, then Thomas Bartholin, and finally, Jean Walæus. But if I except the testimony of Peiresc, of which I do not well see the origin, all the others are but one. For it is Fulgence who in showing the manuscript of Sarpi to Vesling confides to him the secret; it is Vesling who transmitted this secret to Thomas Bartholin, and it is Bartholin who commuicates it to Jean Walæus.

There remain then two distinct pieces of evidence—that of Peiresc and that of Fulgence.

To these two I oppose two others; in the first place, the testimony of Harvey which I have just cited, a man more competent to give evidence upon the question at issue than Peiresc or Fulgence, and in the second place that of Gaspard Bauhin, the immortal author of *Pinax*, like Harvey, a pupil of Fabricius: in his *Traité d'anatomie*, published in 1592, he thus expresses himself; "we find no one who has made mention of these valves before the celebrated Fabricius ab Acquapendente, our master in anatomy, who eighteen years ago, demonstrated them for the first time in the amphitheatre of Padua.[1]

(1) Neminem legimus qui earum fecerit mentionem ante cl. anatomicum Hieronymum Fabricium ab Acquapendente, patavinum, anatomicum præceptorem nostrum, qui ante annos octodecim eas in patavino theatro demonstravit, et ipsimet demonstrari vidimus ab eodem ante annos quatuordecim."—*Anat. lib.* ii.

Morgagni, the most learned historian and at the same time the most careful critic anatomy has ever had, Morgagni knew, examined and weighed all this pretended testimony which is advanced, and the whole of it has not affected his judgment. He concluded, as I have concluded, that the discovery of the valves of the veins was not made by Sarpi but by Fabricius.[1]

Sarpi and the circulation of the blood.

Those who admit these evidences which I have been combatting, so long as they relate to Fabricius, and believe themselves able to reject them when they concern Harvey, are laboring under a singular delusion. The witnesses cannot be separated.

"The discovery of the circulation," says Vesling, "is an invention of Father Paul's, from whom Fabricius also derived the existence of the valves."

"In this century," says Jean Walæus, "the incomparable Paul, Servite, became acquainted with the valves of the veins, afterward publicly demonstrated by the great anatomist Fabricius, and from their disposition he inferred the movement of the blood. Instructed by this Servite, *ab hoc Servitâ edoctus*, the learned William Harvey studied this

(1) See the fifteenth of the Letters of Morgagni upon Valsalva.—(*Epist. anat. duodeviginti ad script. pertinent Valsalvæ.*)

movement farther and published it in his own name."[1]

How can we separate Harvey from Fabricius? And note that while this was written Harvey still lived, and note well, too, that to his honor he had the good sense not to take notice of it. As we have seen before, Riolan was the only one of his adversaries to whom he responded.

When the enemies of Harvey became convinced that he would not reply to them, they ceased their attacks; they became tired of a fruitless warfare. And this same Thomas Bartholin, who, in his letter to Jean Walæus, dated in 1642, revealed the famous secret, wrote some years after, in 1673, as follows:

"In the last century Cæsalpinus divined something of the circulation; but the honor of the first discovery, *laus primæ inventionis*, is due to Harvey, an Englishman. It is true that Father Fulgence found something relating to it in the papers

(1) "Hoc seculo denuò vir incomparabilis Paulus, Servita, venetus, valvularum in venis fabricam observavit accuratius, quam magnus anatomicus Fabricius ab Acquapendente posteà edidit, et ex eà valvularum constitutione aliisque experimentis hunc sanguinis motum deduxit, egrioque scripto asseruit, quod etiamnum intelligo apud venetos asservari .... Ab hoc Servità edoctus vir doctissimus Gulielmus Harvejus sanguinus hunc motum accuratius indagavit, inventis auxit, probavit firmius, et suo divulgavit nomine."—(*De motu chyli et sanguinis*, etc.)

of Paul Sarpi, which has given birth to the conjecture that Sarpi opened the way for Harvey; the fact simply is that Harvey, as I have learned from his friends, was connected with Sarpi and communicated to him his thoughts concerning the movement of the blood, and that the latter took and preserved notes of the subject in his papers, according to his custom. Everybody recognizes Harvey as the author of the discovery."[1]

Here then the tune is changed. In the *letter* of Thomas Bartholin it is from Sarpi that Harvey obtained the discovery; and in the *book* of this same Bartholin it is from Harvey that Sarpi learned what he knew of it. After that rely upon secrets and confidential relations for writing history!

I come now to the new document produced by M. Bianchi-Giovini: it is one of Sarpi's letters. Sarpi was a man of prodigious capacity; he had

(1) "Priori seculo Cæsalpinus aliquid de eâ (de circulatione) divinavit, ... sed clarius nostro seculo innotuit Harvejo, anglo, cui primæ inventionis, promulgationis et per varia argumenta et experimenta probationis, prima laus meritò debetur .... Quamquam P. Fulgentius in schedis Pauli Sarpæ, veneti, aliquid hâc de re invenerit, unde suspicandi orta est occasio Sarpam Harvejo viam monstrasse; sed, sicut ab amicis Harveji accepi, familiaris hic illi fuit, unde cum has de sanguinis motu cogitationes illi communicasset, Sarpa in schedis retulit more suo, posterisque ansam dubitandi subministravit. At Harvejo omnes applaudunt, *circulationis* auctori."—(Thomæ Bartholini, *Anatome*, etc.; *Libell. de venis:* Leyde, 1673.)

that perspicacity which divines all things; he was capable of discovering all things. But this is not a reason that he discovered anything, and we can not therefore agree with the decision of Fulgence.[1]

The following is the letter, or rather the fragment of a letter, for it is but a fragment, but one which is striking from the marks it presents of superior penetration: "As to your exhortations, I should say to you that I am no longer, as formerly, in a position which permits me to charm my leisure hours in making anatomical observations upon lambs, goats, cows and other animals: could I do so, I should be at this time more desirous than ever of repeating some of them, on account of the noble present you have made me of the great and very useful work of the illustrious Vesalius. There is really a great analogy between the things already remarked and noted by me in regard to the movement of the blood in the animal body, and to the structure as well as the use of the valves, and what I find with pleasure indicated, although less clearly, in Book vii., chap. xix. of

(1) "Eâ Sarpius fuit ingenii vi, eo studio, eâ industriâ, solertiâ sagacitate, ut tametsi in omnibus propemodum scientiis atque artibus, non ea omnia quæ ipsi in vitâ istâ (the Life of *Sarpi* by Fulgence) tribuuntur (nihil autem fere non tribuitur) primus deprehendere .... posset."—(Morgagni: xv. *Lettre sur Valsalva.*)

this work. It is to be inferred from what appears there, that by the insufflation of fresh air into the trachea of the dying, or of those in whom the vital functions appear to have ceased, we can succeed in restoring to their blood the movement it has lost and in prolonging life some time. If it is thus, and we can scarcely doubt it after the experiments of this great anatomist, I am more than ever confirmed in the opinion that the air which we respire contains a principle or agent capable of vivifying the sanguineous fluid, and of reëstablishing its movement in those who have been surprised by mortal faintings or asphyxiated by the pernicious vapors which exhale from tombs, ... an agent, in a word, such as is alluded to in the Scriptures, in these words: *anima omnis carnis* (that is to say, of every living thing) *in sanguine est*, of which also many ancient philosophers have spoken, and nearer our own times, Marsile Ficin, Pic de la Mirandole, etc., etc."

Thus writes Sarpi! He knew of the existence of the valves; he meditated upon the movement of the blood; from some experiments of Vesalius upon the insufflation of air into the trachea to maintain the movement of the heart he concluded the presence in the air of a principle vivifying, active, penetrating; a *vital air;* our *oxygen:* he concludes and seems to predict, for all this is original and unpremeditated with him,[1] he predicts the part which this agent, still unknown, will play in animating the movements of the heart when about ceasing, and in restoring the asphyxiated to life. What sagacity, what perspicuity, what penetration, and what power has the human mind in some of the chosen of God!

If in these few lines Sarpi had said to us: "I discovered the valves," in my estimation all would be settled; I would proclaim Sarpi the author of the discovery of the valves; genius has always a right to be believed; but Sarpi contents himself with saying that he knew of them, and that he had at times written some *notes* upon their *structure* and their *use;* and farther, the fragment of the letter in which he speaks of this is evidently posterior to the publication of the discovery of Fabricius.

The fragment is without date; but to me it appears easy to see that it could not have been

(1) In contrast with the studies of Vesalius which were strictly experimental. In order to examine the movements of the heart Vesalius opened the chest, and when he saw life about to be extinguished he restored the animal and kept it alive by artificial respiration .... "Ut verò vita animali quodammodo restituatur, foramen in asperæ arteriæ caudice tentandum est, cui canalis ex calamo aut arundine indetur, isque inflabitur, ut pulmo assurgat, ipsumque animal quodammodo aerem ducat: levi enim inflatu in vivo hoc animali pulmo tantum quanta thoracis erat cavitas intumet, corque vires denuo assumit, et motus ipsus differentia pulchre evariat."—(*Vesalii, De corp. hum. fabr.*, lib. vii., ch. xix.)

written before the demonstration of the valves by Fabricius, and this point will suffice for the present. "I am no longer, as formerly, in a position," etc. says Sarpi. Now if this *formerly* be placed at four or five years, and it is difficult to estimate it at less, Sarpi, who was only twenty-two years old in 1574 when Fabricius publicly demonstrated the valves, could not have been more than seventeen or eighteen at the time when he is said to have discovered them, an age at which little thought is spent on the profound mechanism of the animal body, or on one of the most hidden structures of the organism. The fact is little probable.[1] Sarpi was acquainted with the existence of the valves, but he did not discover them.

(1) But, it may be said, Fabricius himself quotes Sarpi in another place and with great praise. The case is very different; firstly, the observation for which Fabricius quotes Sarpi was not made until much later; secondly, it was made at the suggestion of Fabricius; thirdly, it was not a quotation concerning profound anatomy or hidden stauctures; it was simply in regard to the different action of the *iris* under a strong and under a feeble light. .... "Re igitur cum amico quodam nostro communicatâ ille tandem fortè id observavit, scilicet nonmodo in cato, sed in homine et quocumque animali, foramen uveæ in majori contrahi luce, in minori dilatari. Quod arcanum observatum est, et mihi significatum à Rev. Patre Magistro Paulo veneto, Ordinis ut appellant Servorum Theologo, philosophoque insigni, sed mathematicarum disciplinarum præcipuèque optices, maximè studioso, quem hoc loco honoris gratiâ nomino ...." (*De oculo*, etc., pars 111, cap. vi.

Farther, in regard to the circulation; of that he knew nothing at all.

"There is a grand analogy," says he, "between the things observed and noted by me as to the movement of the blood and the use of the valves, and what I find indicated, although less clearly, in Vesalius." But Vesalius knew nothing of the valves, and of the movement of the blood only that which takes place in the arteries,[1] and he was completely deceived as to the course of the blood in the veins: he says, "the blood is carried into the whole body by the veins."[2] He should have said just the reverse—it is carried into the different parts of the body by the arteries and brought back from them by the veins. If Sarpi understood the true course of the blood, how is it that he did not perceive this error of Vesalius? And if he did perceive it how could he say that there was a great

(1) Galen had plainly proved that the arteries contain blood as we have already shown; but this had been forgotten and it was universally believed in the schools that the arteries only contained *vital spirits*. Vesalius again proved that the arteries contain blood: "atque ita .... observatur in arteriis sanguinem naturâ contineri, si quando arteriam in vivis aperimus."—(*De corp. hum. fabr.*, p. 568.)

(2) "Ceterum in venarum usu inquirendo, vix quoque vivorum sectione opus est: quum in mortuis affatim discamus eas sanguinem per universum corpus deferre, et partem aliquam non nutriri in quâ insignis vena in vulneribus præscinditur." —(*Ibid.*)

analogy between the ideas of Vesalius and his own? His ideas were no more advanced nor any more correct than those of Vesalius.

There is just cause for surprise here. For while Sarpi wrote at Padua these uncertain lines in regard to the circulation, Cæsalpinus wrote at Pisa this sentence so precise and so clear: "The blood conducted to the heart by the veins receives there its last perfection, and this perfection acquired it is carried by the arteries to the whole body."[1]

Once again, then, could the *circulation* be better understood and defined? The true predecessor of Harvey was not Sarpi but Cæsalpinus, and there is nothing to conceal about it; the secret may be revealed to the whole world.

Harvey and the true use of the valves.

Fabricius did not see the use of the valves. He believed that they only served to prevent the too great distension of the thin coats of the veins:[2] it

(1) "In animalibus videmus alimentum per venas duci ad cor tanquam ad officinam caloris insiti, et, adepta inibi ultimâ perfectione, per arterias in universum corpus distribui."—(*De plantis*, lib. i., cap. ii., p. 3, Florence, 1583.)

(2) .... "Dicere procul dubio tutò possumus ad prohibendam quoque venarum distensionem fuisse ostiola à Summo Opifice fabrefacta: distendi autem ac dilatari facile potuissent venæ, cum ex membranosâ substantiâ eâque simplici ac tenui sint conflatæ ...." (Fabr. ab Acquap: *De venarum ostiolis.*)

is for this reason, he says, that the arteries, having very thick coats, do not have valves.[1]

Harvey was perfectly right, then, when he said that nobody before him, Harvey, had known the the use of the *valves*.[2] Upon this point it is necessary to read and re-read all his thirteenth chapter, which is the chapter of his genius. Fabricius, who believed that the blood ran from the heart to the extremities in the veins, concluded that the use of the valves was to moderate its current, and prevent its pouring into the inferior veins, accumulating there, distending them, etc., etc.

You do not see all the import of your discovery, Harvey says to him; you believe that the valves limit themselves to moderating the course of the

(1) "Arteriis autem ostiola non fuere necessaria, neque ad distensionem prohibendam propter tunicæ crassitiem ac robur ...." (*Ibid.*)

(2) "Harum valvularum usum inventor non est assecutus, neque alii, qui dixerunt, ne pondere deorsum sanguis in inferiora subitò ruat. Sunt namque in jugularibus deorsum spectantes, et sanguinem sursum prohibentes ferri: nam ubique spectant à radicibus venarum versus cordis locum ...." (*Exercit. anatom. de mortu cordis*, etc. cap. xiii.) "If you attempt," says Fabricius, "to force the blood downward you will plainly see it arrested in its course by the veins, and by no other means was I conducted to their discovery: Si enim premere, aut deorsum fricando adigere sanguinem per venas tentes, cursum istius ab ipsis ostiolis intercipi, remorarique aperte videbis: neque enim aliter ego in hujusmodi notitiam sum deductus."—(*De venarum ostiolis.*)

blood; they do much more, they oppose themselves completely to any flow in the direction you suppose, and compel it to pursue an opposite course. Remark, I pray you, that they are all directed toward the heart; they constrain the blood, then, to flow always toward the heart,[1] to turn toward itself, to return to the point from which it set out; to flow back by the veins to the heart from which it came by the arteries.

That is the circulation, Fabricius, and it is the valves that demonstrate it.

Harvey and his predecessors.

The predecessors of Harvey are Fabricius, who discovered the *valves*, and Cæsalpinus, who so well described the *general circulation;*[2] this same Cæsalpinus, who not less clearly described the *pulmonary circulation;*[3] and Realdo Columbus, who

(1) "......... Adeo ut venæ patentes et apertæ sint regredienti sanguini ad cor, progredienti vero a corde omnino occlusæ."—(*Exercit. anat. de mortu. cordis*, etc., cap. xii.)

(2) See page 29 for the proof of his having been the first to call attention to the swelling of the veins *below* a ligature.

(3) "Idcircò pulmo per venam arteriis similem ex dextro cordis ventriculo fervidum hauriens sanguinem, eumque per anastomosim arteriæ venali reddens, quâ in sinistrum cordis ventriculum tendit, transmisso interim aere frigido per asperæ arteriæ canales, qui juxtà arteriam venalem protenduntur, non tamen osculis communicantes, ut putavit Galenus, solo tactu temperat. Huic sanguinis *circulationi* ex dextro

saw the pulmonary circulation before Cæsalpinus, and Servetus who saw it before Columbus.

Nemesius, bishop of Emesa.

I limit myself here to the consideration of two or three points already developed in the preceding chapters.

It is certain that Servetus discovered the pulmonary circulation; but it is equally certain that the absurd book in which this beautiful discovery was published, was burned almost as soon as it was printed. Servetus did not influence any of his successors.

In the order of dates, then, Columbus is the first; then comes Cæsalpinus, then Fabricius and then Harvey.

It has been said that Servetus might have derived some assistance from Nemesius, bishop of Emesa.[1] It is a mistake. Servetus did not influence any one, nor did any one influence him.

cordis ventriculo per pulmones in sinistrum ejusdem ventriculum optimè respondent ea quæ ex dissectione apparent. Nam duo sunt vasa in dextrum ventriculum desinentia, duo etiam in sinistrum: duorum autem unum intromittit tantum, alterum educit, membranis eo ingenio constitutis."—(*Quæst. perpatetica*, lib. v., cap. iv.)

(1) "......... These views he might possibly have borrowed from a work of Nemesius, entitled *De natura hominis* .... This bishop explains the phenomena of the circulation of the blood like Servetus."—(*Biog. univ. art. Servet.*)

Nemesius did not say a word upon the pulmonary circulation, so clearly explained by Servetus; he spoke of the *pulse*, of *animal heat*, of the *vital spirits*, and wrote of all of them as Galen wrote. He followed Galen in everything.[1] The chief merit

(1) "Pulsuum motus, qui vitalis facultas dicitur, initium habet à corde, et maximè à sinistro ejus ventriculo, qui spirabilis appellatur, et innatum vitalemque calorem omni parti corporis per arterias, ut jecur alimentum per venas, impertit. .... Nam spiritus vitalis ab eo per arterias in totum corpus dispergitur. Plerumque autem inter se hæc tria simul finduntur: vena, arteria, nervus, e tribus initiis quæ animal gubernant profecta. E cerebro, principio movendi et sentiendi, nervus. E jecore, principio sanguinis et alentis facultatis, vena, vas sanguinis. E corde, principio vitalis facultatis, arteria, vas spiritus. Cum autem hæc coeunt, mutuis inter se commodis fruuntur. Vena enim pastum suppeditat nervis et arteriæ. Arteria venæ calorem naturalem et spiritum vitalem impertit. Unde neque arteria inveniri potest sine tenui sanguine, neque vena sine spiritu, qui ad vaporis naturam accedat. Diducitur autem vehementer, et contrahitur arteria, harmoniâ quâdam, et ratione, initio motus à corde sumpto. Sed dum diducitur, à proximis venis vi trahit tenuem sanguinem, cujus respiratio fit alimentum spiritui vitali. Dum autem contrahitur, quod in se fuliginosi est per totum corpus et occulta foramina exhaurit, quomodo cor, per os, et nares, quidquid fuliginosi est, expirando sursum expellit." This is all that Nemesius has said. This *pulse*, which derives its power from the heart—this *vital heat*, which has its origin in the left ventricle—these *arteries* which carry that vital heat throughout the body—these *veins* which distribute the *aliment*, taking it always from the *liver*—this *tripod* of life, the *brain*, the *heart* and the *liver*,—all this is derived from Galen, as we have already shown. One or two lines seem to point to a

of Servetus is that he did not follow Galen but contradicted him, that he saw differently from Galen and saw well. "If any one will compare," (he says with confidence,) "these things with what Galen has written in Books vi. and vii. of his *Usage of Parts*, he will comprehend the truth which Galen did not perceive."

It is not worth while to deprive a man who has had the misfortune to be burned, and to be burned for an absurd book, of the signal honor of having been the first to depart from Galen, to think for himself, and to originate a discovery which was, it is true, but an incomplete view, yet an incomplete view of phenomena the entire comprehension of which has sufficed to immortalize the name of Harvey.

communication between the veins and the arteries, "Sed dum diducitur (arteria) à proximis venis vi trahit sanguinem .... Unde neque arteria inveniri potest sine tenui sanguine, neque vena sine spiritu ...." But is this a comprehensible mechanism? Putting aside, too, the liver distributing aliment to all parts by the veins: "Jecur alimentum per venas impertit, etc., etc."

V.

SERVETUS AND THE FORMATION OF THE SPIRITS.

Servetus discovered the pulmonary circulation. The fact is clear. I have already quoted the beautiful, the immortal passage in which he has described it much better than was done several years after him by Columbus and Cæsalpinus. Leibnitz justly alludes to Cæsalpinus in these words: "Andrew Cæsalpinus, physician, an author of merit, and who approached nearest to the discovery of the circulation of the blood after Michael Servetus."

There are two things here which surprise us. How Servetus, elsewhere so confused, could be so admirably lucid in a few pages. And, how a discovery in physiology, in pure and profound physiology, should be found in a book having for its title "The Restitution of Christianity."[1]

I had for a long time desired to enlighten myself upon the latter point. The kindness of my friend and learned *confrere* of the Institute, M. Magnin,[2] finally furnished me the opportunity. I have seen, I have touched the book of Servetus. A copy of

(1) For the entire title of this work, see note 1, page 22.

(2) One of the conservators of the Imperial Library.

this famous work is carefully preserved in our library, and to complete all, this copy, the only one perhaps now in existence, belonged to Colladon, one of the accusers raised up by the pitiless Calvin against the unfortunate Servetus. It formerly belonged to the English physician, Richard Mead, celebrated for his treatise on poisons. Mead gave it to de Boze. It was afterwards purchased by the Royal Library at a very high price. In it Colladon has underscored the passages upon which he accused Servetus. Finally, and as a last mark of undeniable authority, several pages of this unlucky volume are scorched and blackened by fire. It was not saved from the pile where author and work were burned together until after the conflagration had commenced!

Let us turn aside from these frightful *souvenirs*. We are only occupied here, thank God, with physiology.

I must commence by informing those who are carried away by their zeal for Harvey, and go so far as to suggest that the passage concerning the pulmonary circulation must have been intercalated, that they are mistaken. There is no intercalation, no interpolation, no trickery. The passage belongs entirely to Servetus, and nothing remains but to submit. A long time before Harvey there was a man of genius occupied with this great subject of the circulation of the blood, and that man was Servetus.

But how has Servetus managed to thrust a description of the *pulmonary circulation* into a work on the *Restitution of Christianity?*

When we cast a glance over the writings of Servetus, which I aver I have not done until now, we soon perceive what part he took in theology; he attached himself singly and obstinately to the literal sense. He sought every where for the literal meaning; he accused everybody, and above all Calvin, of not understanding it; he accumulated quotations to prove that he alone comprehended it.

It is not necessary to leave the subject before us to find an example. The Scriptures say that the soul is in the blood, that the soul is the blood itself; *anima est in sanguine; anima ipsa est sanguis.*

Since the soul is in the blood, says Servetus, to know how the soul is formed it is necessary to know how the blood is formed, and to learn this we must see how it moves; and it is thus that in writing on the *restitution of christianity* he is conducted to the formation of the soul, and from the formation of the soul to that of the blood, and from this to the pulmonary circulation.

But this is not all. From this same blood, which furnishes the soul, the *spirits* are also formed. Servetus explains successively the formation of the *blood*, of the *spirits*, and of the *soul*, and from all this there results a philosophy half of which is theological, half physiological, extremely singular from beginning to end, and which he calls *divine*.

"In order that you may have, dear reader," he says, "a complete explanation of the soul and the spirits, I will add here a divine philosophy which you will easily understand, if you have applied yourself to anatomy."[1]

He then commences to explain the formation of the *spirits*. We have already seen what were Galen's theories of their formation. Servetus did not cite Galen but he copied him. He quoted and criticised a certain Aphrodisæus, a physician who lived at the commencement of the sixteenth century. Aphrodisæus, he says, reckons three kinds of spirits, the natural, the vital and the animal; but there are not three kinds, there are only two, the vital and animal.[2] The *natural* are the same as

(1) "Ut vero totam animæ et spiritus rationem habeas, lector, divinam hic philosophiam adjungam, quam facile intelliges, si in anatome fueris exercitatus."

(2) "Tres spiritus vocat Aphrodisæus, naturalis, vitalis et animalis......... Vere non sunt tres, sed duo spiritus distincti."

the *vital.* The vital spirits pass from the arteries into the veins and are there called natural.[1]

There are thus three principles: the *blood*, the seat of which is the liver and the veins of the body, the *vital spirits*, which are in the heart and arteries, and the *animal spirits*, situated in the brain and in the nerves.[2]

It is from the blood contained in the liver that the soul draws its first material by an admirable elaboration;[3] and for this reason the soul is said *to be in the blood, to be the blood itself*, that is to say, the *spirit of the blood.*[4]

But we must learn first how the *vital spirits* are formed. They are formed by the mixture of air, drawn in by respiration, with the blood which the right ventricle sends to the left, a mixture which

(1) "Vitalis est spiritus qui per anastomoses ab arteriis communicatur venis, in quibus dicitur naturalis."

(2) Primus ergo est sanguinis, cujus sedes est in hepate et corporis venis. Secundus est spiritus vitalis, cujus sedes est in corde et corporis arteriis. Tertius est spiritus animalis, cujus sedes est in cerebro et corporis nervis.

(3) Ex hepatis sanguine est animæ materia per elaborationem mirabilem.

(4) Hinc dicitur anima esse in sanguine, et anima ipsa esse sanguis, id est spiritus sanguineus......Non dicitur anima principaliter esse in parietibus cordis, aut in corpore ipso cerebri, aut hepatis, sed in sanguine, ut docet ipse Deus: *Genes.* 9, *Lev.* 17 *et Deut.* 12.

takes place in the lungs; for it is not necessary to believe as is commonly taught, says Servetus, that the blood passes from one ventricle to the other through the medium septum; it can only pass from one ventricle to the other by way of the lungs;[1] and here comes in that singular passage on the pulmonary circulation.

I have already quoted and already translated the whole of this remarkable passage. I content myself with alluding to it here, and must return alas! to blind Servetus—to Servetus confused, and absurd, no longer inspired by genius.

The *vital spirits*, formed in the lungs, pass thence into the left ventricle and from there into the arteries, in such a manner, however, that the particles of greatest rarity tend always upwards, and becoming more and more elaborated, arrive at the *plexus retiformis*, situated at the base of the brain, where from *vital* the spirits commence to change into *animal*.[2] Finally, by a further and

(1) Ad quam rem est prius intelligenda substantialis generatio ipsius vitalis spiritus qui ex aere inspirato et subtilissimo sanguine componitur... Generatur exfacta in pulmonibu mixtione inspirati aeris cum elaborato sanguine, quem dexter ventriculis cordis sinistro communicat...... Fit autem communicatio hæc, non parietem cordis medium, ut vulgo creditur, sed magno artificio a dextro cordis ventriculo, longo per pulmones ductu, agitatur sanguis subtilis......

(2) "Ille itaque spiritus vitalis a sinistro cordis ventriculo in arterias totius corporis deinde transfunditur, ita ut qui

complete elaboration the *animal spirits* pass from the *retiform plexus* into the *choroid plexus*, and it is in these little arteries that the soul resides[1]

I omit, for I am in haste to finish, a host of anatomical errors which Servetus joined to his confused reasonings, and which besides are only the anatomical and physiological errors of the times in which he lived, such for instance as the brain being without any peculiar function but only serving as a pillar or cushion for the vessels of the *animal spirits* ;[2] that the nerves are the continuation of the arteries and constitute a third order of vessels ;[3] that the ventricles of the brain communicate with the nasal fossæ by the foraminæ of

tenuior est superiora petat, ubi magis adhuc elaboratur, præcipue in plexu retiformi, sub basi cerebri sito, in quo ex vitali fieri incipit animalis, ad propriam rationalis animæ sedem accedens."

(1) Iterum ille (spiritus animalis) fortius mentis igneâ vi tenuatur, elaboratur, et perficitur, in tenuissimis vasis, seu capillaribus arteriis, quæ in plexibus choroidibus sitæ sunt, et ipsissimam mentem continent.

(2) Ex his satis constat, mollem illam cerebri massam non propriè esse rationalis animæ sedem, cum frigida sit et sensus expers, sed esse veluti pulvinum dictorum vasorum ne rumpantur, et custodem animalis spiritus......

(3) Vasa illa miraculo magno tenuissime contexta, tametsi arteriæ dicantur, sunt tamen fines arteriarum, tendentes ad originem nervorem, ministerio meningum. Est novum quoddam genus vasorum......

the ethmoid bone, a pretended communication in which Servetus saw a great advantage, for, in the first place, the external air penetrates thus to the soul and ventilates and replenishes it,[1] and in the second place, the soul gets rid, through these openings, of mucus which would have embarrassed its action,[2] and also escapes a very great peril, for the evil spirit, *spiritus nequam*, which in its nature resembles air, enters sometimes by the same route, by these same openings in the ethmoid bone, and reaching the ventricles of the brain, fights there incessantly against the soul and holds it beseiged until the light of God appears and puts it to fight, etc., etc.[3]

I leave Servetus; but I avail myself of the opportunity which his doctrines have given me, to

(1)...... Facti sunt ventriculi ut ad spatia eorum inania penetrans per ossa ethmoïde inspirati aeris portio......animalem intus contentum spiritum reficiat, et animam ventilet.

(2) ....Facti sunt ventriculi illi ad expurgamenta cerebri recipienda, veluti cloacæ, ut probant excrementa ibi recepta, et meatus ad palatum et nares... Et quandò ventriculi oplentur pituitâ, ut arteriæ ipsæ choroïdis eâ immergantur, tum subitò generatur apoplexia.

(3) Spiritus nequam, cujus potestas est aeris, unà cum inspirato à nobis aere, lacunas illas liberè ingreditur, ut ubi cum spiritu nostro, intra vasa illa, velut in arce collocato, jugiter, dimicat. Imò eum ita undique obsidet, ut vix illi liceat respirare, nisi quum superveniens lux spiritus Dei malum spiritum fugat.

cast a rapid glance at the long reign of *spirits* in physiology.

The spirits played in ancient physiology the same part which is filled now by *properties*, or rather the *forces*. Hence their great importance. Galen explained everything by means of the *spirits;* and, as we have seen, he gave three species of them, natural, vital and animal.

So much for antiquity. Reckoning from the revival of letters, Galen's three kinds of spirits were revived and existed up to the time of Descartes. When Descartes came he took a fancy for the *animal spirits* and rejected the others.

I have already quoted this paragraph from Bordeu: "The ancients admitted three kinds of spirits; it is not easy to understand by what fatality the natural and the vital have been unable to maintain themselves and have succumbed, while the animal have survived.[1]" I have already responded that Bordeu had not paid attention, and that nothing is easier to understand. The natural and vital spirits gave way because Descartes excluded them; the animal spirits remained because Descartes adopted them. And it is always thus. It is the writer who makes the fortune of words.

Descartes, the powerful renovater of ideas, but

(1) Rech. anat. sur la position des glandes et leur action. § 34.

who borrowed nevertheless, a great deal from the ancients, combined the theory of the *spirits*, which he took from Galen, with the *circulation of the blood* which Harvey had just discovered. He was the first Frenchman who fully understood and clearly described this great phenomenon.

"All those," says, Descartes, "whom the authority of the ancients has not entirely blinded, and who have been willing to open their eyes for the examination of the doctrines of Harvey touching the circulation of the blood, do not doubt that all the veins and the arteries of the body are only channels through which the blood runs unceasingly, taking its course from the right cavity of the heart by the arterial vein, the branches of which are distributed throughout the lungs, and joined to those of the venous artery, through which it passes from the lung into the left side of the heart; then, from there it goes into the grand artery of which the branches, scattered throughout the body, are united to the branches of the vena cava, which return the same blood to the same right cavity of the heart."[1]

The complete phenomena of the circulation of the blood, both general and pulmonary, could not be more completely or more briefly described.

But on the other hand, this is how Descartes

(1) *Les passions de l'âme*: 1re partie, art. 7.

came to conceive of the *animal spirits* and to form his idea in regard to their action in the organs.

"It is known," he says, "that all the movements of the muscles, as well as all the senses, depend upon the nerves, which are like little threads or little tubes coming from the brain, and like it, containing a certain gas or air, very subtile, called the *animal spirits*."[1] . . . .
The most subtile parts of the blood form the animal spirits; and they have no need of receiving for this purpose, any other change in the brain, but are only separated from other and less-refined parts of the blood; for what I call here spirits are only bodies, and have no peculiar properties except that they are extremely small, and they move very quickly like the sparks of fire from a torch, and in such a manner that they do not stop anywhere, but as fast as some enter the cavities of the brain others come out through the pores of its substance, which pores conduct them into the nerves, and from them they pass into the muscles, by which means the body is moved in all the diverse manners of which it is capable of being moved."[2]

What was especially valuable to Descartes in these animal spirits, was that they permitted him

(1) *Les passions de l'âme:* 1re partie, art. 7.

(2) *Ibid*, art. 10.

to explain all the actions of the body without any assistance from the soul; the great and final object of his beautiful philosophy.

"All the movements which we make," he continues, "without our will causing them, as it often happens that we walk, or eat, or indeed perform any of the actions common to us and to the beasts, depend only on the conformation of our members and on the course which the spirits, excited by the heat of the heart, follow naturally in the brain, in the nerves, and in the muscles; in the same manner as the movement of a watch is produced by the force of its spring and the figure of its wheels."[1]

Thus Descartes accounted, by the *course of the spirits* alone, for all the functions of the body; and that being done he arrived at this principal conclusion, viz: "there remains nothing in us which we should attribute to the soul, except our thoughts."[2]

After the first Descartes the philosopher who made the most use of the *spirits*, is one who may be called the second Descartes, Malebranche.

Malebranche commences one of his chapters thus: "Every one knows that the animal spirits are only the most subtile and most agitated parts of the blood, which are produced principally by fermentation and by the violent movement of the muscles which compose the heart, that these spirits are

(1) *Les passions de l'âme:* 1re partie, art. 16.

(2) *Ibid.*, art. 17.

conducted by the arteries with the rest of the blood, as far as the brain . . . . ."[1]

Malebranche conducted the spirits intrepidly, as we see, to the brain; but, having arrived there, how are they separated from that organ? He admitted with good grace that he knew nothing about it. "They are separated from it," he says, "by some parts destined for that purpose, which are not yet known." He explains in another place the difference which he considers to exist between the *animal spirits* and the brain. "There is this difference between the animal spirits and the substance of the brain, the spirits are very restless and very fluid, and the substance of the brain has some solidity and consistence, so that the spirits divide into small parties and disperse in a few hours by transpiring through the pores of the vessels which contain them, and often others come in their place which are not at all similar to them."[2] And Malebranche says, that from this change of spirits arise our changes in humor or temper according to the *different kinds of food and drink* we have used!

"Wine is so spirituous that it is almost wholly formed into animal spirits, but spirits which are libertine, and will not submit themselves readily

(1) *De la Recherche de la verite,* 1st part of book ii., chap. ii .

(2) *Ibid.,* liv. ii., chap. vi.

to the orders of the will, because of their subtility and their excessive agitation. Thus, in the most strong and vigorous men it produces more and greater changes in the imagination and in all parts of the body than food, or than any other beverage. It *trips up one's heels*, as Plautus says; and produces in the mind effects which are not so advantageous as those which Horace describes in the lines commencing—

'Quid non ebrietas designat.' [1]

The great Bossuet, of whom it can scarcely be said that he followed any one in any department of knowledge, nevertheless adopted the ideas of Descartes in philosophy: he says, "the spirits, carried into the muscles by the nerves distributed through the members cause the progressive movements . . . . ."[2] Again, "the spirits are the most lively and most agitated part of the blood, and set in action all the members."[3] "As soon as the spirits are lacking the springs fail for want of a prime mover."[4] "The passions," he says finally, "regarding them solely in the body, seem to be nothing but an extraordinary agitation of the

(1) *De la Recherche de la Verite*, liv. ii., chap. ii.

(2) *De la Connaissance de Dieu et de soi-méme*, chap. ii., § 6.

(3) *Ibid.*, § 9.

(4) *Ibid.*, § 12.

spirits, occasioned by certain objects which we must flee or pursue, etc., etc."[1]

Malebranche died in 1715; Fontenelle in 1757, and with the latter the last superior representative of Cartesianism. With Cartesianism fell the *animal spirits.*

In 1742, a young man full of spirit, full of fire, full of ambition, and having all the audacity of youth, sustained a thesis at the school of Montpelier, in which he arraigned the spirits, attacked them rudely and violently, and what is worse, for all must be told, he ridiculed them.

"Might not an unprejudiced man," he says, "who would give himself the trouble to examine, be able to prove that the existence of any one of these three kinds of spirits—this *tripod*, or if you will, this *triumvirate* of ancient physiology—is but poorly established. As to the manner in which the moderns sustain them, we are struck, first, by the prodigious number of forms which are given to them; some say they are *air*, others that they are *fire*, or *water*, or *lymph;* they are said to be *acid, sulphurous, active, passive;* two or three species of them are given which flow in the same nerves; finally they have received all kinds of figure, even to that of *eddies* or *whirlpools*, or *little balloons with springs*, (*petits ballons á ressort*) to use the terms of

(1) *De la connaisance de Dieu et de soi-méme.*

M. Lieutaud, who is as well persuaded of the existence of these '*ballons*' as he is of the structure which he supposes the brain to have. Let us add, he continues, and always very ingeniously and very judiciously, "let us add that those who admit the existence of the spirits are as much embarrassed to explain the functions of the nerves as those who do not believe in them. Are we any farther advanced after following the infinite details of Boerhaeve and his commentators upon this question? Would it not be better to abandon it once for all, and place it among those tiresome questions with which the ancients commenced their physiologies? Shall we never profit by the errors of those who have preceded us?"

This is the way in which the young Bordeu, then scarcely twenty years old,[1] treated the *spirits*, and such is the fortune of the most beautiful doctrines of philosophy. These same spirits, so deeply revered by all the ancients, and in modern times by such men as Descartes, Bossuet, and Malebranche, end by becoming the convenient subject for the familiar pleasantries of a school-boy.

(1) He was, in truth, just twenty, having been born in 1722, and he presented his thesis in 1742, *Dissertatio physiologica de sensu generice considerato*; but he was thirty when he published, in 1752, his *Recherches anatomique sur la position des glandes et sur leur action;* an excellent and much better matured work, in which he reproduced his criticism of the *spirits*, and from which I have taken the passages just quoted.

After Bordeu came Barthez. Physiology was assuming a new aspect. Barthez, a metaphysician of a superior order, was the first who in physiology formed a clear conception of the forces, I mean of forces arising from the facts, or as he well-called them *experimental causes:*[1] "We can give," he says, "to these general causes (of the phenomena of life,) which I call experimental, and which are only known by their laws which experiment teaches, the synonymous and equally indeterminate names of principles, powers, forces, faculties, etc." "Good method in philosophizing in the science of man requires that there should be referred to a single principle of life in the human body the vital forces which reside in each organ, and which cause its functions, as well general, such as sensibility, nutrition, etc., as special, such as digestion, menstruation, etc."[2]

Meanwhile the true idea of the *experimental cause*, or *principle*, or *force* in physiology was not yet fully developed. Barthez rightly called *forces* the cause of the functions; he was right in his attempt to connect all the secondary forces to one primary, which is the general vital force; but he was wrong to make this general and common force

(1) *Nouv. elem. de la Sc. de l'homme*, Paris, 1806; t. i., *Disc. prelim.*

(2) *Ibid.*

of life an individual being, abstracted and detached from the organs; and he was still farther wrong in believing himself able to explain any particular phenomenon whatever by pronouncing the words *vital principle*, and referring its origin to that, for being necessarily involved in all, the vital principle could not serve as an explanation for any single one.

The true problem is to arrive at the particular force of each particular phenomenon; at the *property* or *peculiar faculty* which causes it. This has been the aim of all physiologists since Haller. Since, by his beautiful experiments, Haller localized irritability in the muscles and sensibility in the nerves, the way for great discoveries and certain advances in physiology has been open, for all physiology is, I would say, in the precise localization of each given vital force in a distinct organic element.

As to the word *spirits*, (for, as soon as the true name of the *causes* was found, it has been only a word,) excluded from science by the railleries of Bordeu, by the high metaphysics of Barthez, and by the positive researches of Haller, it has appeared no more.

Toward the end of the eighteenth century, in 1779, I find it again employed, and perhaps it is the last time it has been used, in a fine page of Buffon's, but it is in a very general sense, and it retains scarcely anything of its primitive and technical meaning. Buffon says, in regard to the indefatigable activity of the smallest birds: "The most substantial nourishment is necessary to support the prodigious vivacity of the humming-bird, compared with its extreme smallness; it may well need a supply of organic molecules to sustain so much strength in such delicate organs, and maintain the expenditure of *spirits* necessary for such perpetual and rapid movements."[1]

(1) *Histoire des oiseaux-mouches.*

VI.

GUY-PATIN AND THE CONTEST BETWEEN ANCIENT AND MODERN PHYSIOLOGY.

The *Letters* of Guy-Patin reveal to us a very curious epoch in the history of the Faculty of Medicine of Paris, and even in that of the science itself. I reckon three grand eras in medicine since the revival of letters: the Arabian, the Greek and Latin, and the modern, which commences with the discovery of the circulation of the blood.

The era which Guy-Patin pictures for us is the second of these three divisions, the Greek and Latin epoch, which may be called the *erudite* period of French medicine. The yoke of the Arabians had been thrown of; Hippocrates, Aristotle, Galen, those masters of ancient learning, were studied with enthusiasm, and everything modern was despised—the circulation of the blood, the lymphatics, chemistry, and everything else.

Guy-Patin was, *par excellence*, the man of this period:[1] he combatted the Arabians; he denounced

(1) Although coming a little later. The discovery of the circulation of the blood dates between 1619 and 1628, and the first letters of Guy-Patin were written in 1630. He belonged by his birth to the third epoch, and by his doctrines to the second.

the moderns, he was fanatically devoted to Hippocrates and Galen; he would receive neither the circulation of the blood nor chemistry, which certainly are not to be found in Galen or in Hippocrates; finally, to these medical prejudices he added two others, he hated *antimony* because it was the gift of the chemists and *cinchona* because it was introduced by the Jesuits.

The best work of the period under examination, the age of Guy-Patin, of Riolan, of Baillou and of Fernel, was the simplification of medicine and particularly of therapeutics. The therapeutics of the Arabians was a chaos. The Greeks did not use enough remedies—the Arabians multiplied them without limit. There was everything in their therapeia: alchemy, and astrology, while *occult qualities* predominated. A certain boldness of spirit was necessary to clear science of these false surroundings. Fernel, the first physician of his time, still believed in astrology.[1] We must pay great attention, he says, to astrological observations: *Astrologica etiam observatio ut non parum efficax tenenda.*[2] We read in Guy de Chauliac

(1) He at least commenced by believing it; he regretted afterwards the time employed in it. See his biography by Plancy: *Joannis Fernelii, Ambiani, Galliarum archiatri,* UNIVERSA MEDICINA, *etc., Genevæ,* 1680.

(2) *Ibid., De venæ sectione,* lib. ii. cap, xiv p. 202.

that the figure of a lion imprinted in gold, cured pains in the loins.[1]

Guy-Patin admired Fernel; he called him, and with justice, a *great man:* "I esteem him as the wisest and most polished of the moderns;"[2] nevertheless he did not join him in his belief in astrology and *occult qualities.*

"I do not believe," he says, "in occult qualities in medicine, whatever Fernel and others may have said on the subject, for their sayings are not all scripture truth. In fact, I believe in medicine only what I see . . . . . Fernel was a great man, ... but, as he did not say everything, so also he has not said everything truly, in his writings; and if the good man, who is too soon dead, to our great sorrow, had lived longer, he would undoubtedly have changed some things in his works, and especially upon this point."[3]

He says elsewhere in regard to Jacques Charpentier and his commentary on Alcinous: "He

(1) Astruc: *Memoirs pour servir a l'histoire de la Faculte de medicine de Montpellier*, Paris, 1767, p. 191.

(2) *Letters de Guy-Patin*, nouvelle edition augmentee de letters inéditees, précédées d'une Notice biographique, accompagnée de remarques scientifiques, historiques, et literaires, par Reveillé-Parise, 1846, t i, p. 10.

(3) *Ibid*, t. i, p. 9.

[The quotations from Guy-Patin occurring hereafter are from his "Letters" unless otherwise indicated.—*Tr.*]

there follows particularly the guidance and the opinion of Fernel, who in these matters was a great Platonist, and who believed much more than I do of demonomania."

In truth, Guy-Patin could scarcely be reproached with being too credulous. I speak, of course, only in regard to medicine, and I think that this sentence of Bayle applies well to him; "his creed was not burdened with many articles."[1]

His creed contained indeed so few articles that there were only two of them: *bleeding* and *purging!* All the rest, antimony, opium, tea, cinchona, etc., are rejected; *opium* as a *poison*, *tea* as "an impertinent novelty of the age," *antimony* because it was proscribed by the faculty, and *cinchona*, worse than all, because it was the *Jesuit's powder!*[2]

Of all the new remedies Guy-Patin was alone favorable to *senna;* but, in revenge, to that he was entirely devoted. He says; "senna works more miracles than all the drugs brought to us from the Indies." He added to senna, cassia, and the syrup of white roses; and that was his entire pharmacopeia. "So long as we have senna, cassia, and syrup of white roses, we can continue to deliver Paris from the tyranny of the apothecaries."

(1) *Dict. hist. et critique* art. Guy-Patin.

(2) *Letters*, tt. i and ii.

This man with a mind so active, so penetrating and so prompt, but at the same time so prejudiced, so determined, and so self-willed, imposed upon himself the task of simplifying the science of medicine, of rendering it *easy* and *familiar;*[1] I make use of his own expressions. For he saw it everywhere disgraced by the superstitious practices[2] of the Arabians, by the covetousness of the apothecaries, and by the blind tenacity of the chemical physicians of his time. He assisted Guenaut in his experiments with *antimony*, experiments which were often fatal, if we may believe Guy-Patin, or even the poet, which is the same as to say all the world.

According to Guy-Patin antimony alone has killed more people than did the King of Sweden in Germany; and everybody knows what the poet says:

> "On compterait plutôt combien dans un printemps
> Guenaut et l'antimoine ont fait mourir de gens......"[3]

After this we need not be astonished at the war which Guy-Patin carried on against the Arabians, against antimony, and against apothecaries; against the *apothecaries* above all, for them in he could par-

(1) "Je rends la pharmacie la plus populaire qu'il m' est possible." (T. i, p. 23.)

(2) "It is the Arabians who have introduced into medicine these scrupulous and superstitious observances." (t. ii, p. 68.)

(3) Boilean: *Satire*, iv.

don nothing; neither their *Arabianism*, their *chemistry*, their *drugs*, nor their *pills?*

"He also spoke to me of M. Moze, the apothecary, who esteems me highly as he says; upon which I expressed my astonishment, in view of the fact that I had never done anything to make the apothecaries esteem me, that I had never prescribed their *bezoars*, nor their *cordial waters*, neither *theriaca*, nor *mithridate*, neither the *confection* of *hyacinth* nor of *alkermes*, nor the *powder of vipers*, nor *antimonial wine*, nor *pearls*, nor *precious stones*, nor any other such Arabian follies; that I always preferred simple remedies which were neither dear nor rare, and that I made the science of medicine as simple as I possibly could."

"As to my dear enemies, the apothecaries," he says again, "they have complained to our faculty of my last thesis in which they are ridiculed. . . . . I spoke against their *bezoars*, their *confection of alkermes*, their *theriaque*, and their *charges*." . . . . . . "I leave this multitude of remedies to those who practice medicine for pomp and display, and who have an understanding with the apothecaries." [1]

(1) *Letters*, t. iii, p. 541. "The apothecaries are enraged against those physicians who, to prevent their tyranny, prescribe in French and make their own remedies: cassia, senna, syrup of peach flowers, of white roses, and of chicory with rhubarb, suffice for nearly everything. I have never seen a

Thus then even in his most lively pleasantries at the expense of his "dear enemies the apothecaries," Guy-Patin never forgot the object he had in view, the philosophic and elevated idea of simplifying medicine. "For myself, I agree with MM. les Pietres, whose motto is—*ad bene medendum, quam pauca, sed selecta et bene probata remedia.*" "The grand Chancellor of England, Lord Bacon, has wisely said that *multitudo remediorum est filia ignorantiæ.*"

But by constantly laboring to impress this view he exaggerated its importance; his only remedies, as I just now said, were cathartics and phlebotomy, and by a sort of compensation, upon his side, he abused them.

Let us commence with the latter. He ordered bleeding at every period of life, in infancy as well as old age;[1] he bled a patient *thirty-two times* during one illness; he caused himself to be bled *seven times* for a cold; he bled his mother-in-law who was eighty-years of age, *four times;* he or-

disease curable at all, which could not be cured without antimony, although sometimes for the benefit of the most bigoted, I make use of our confections *scammonées* such as *diaphenic, diaprun solutif, diacartheme, dipsilium*; but we must watch closely and not take *martre pour renard.*'

(1) "We cure our patients who are past eighty by bleeding, and we deplete as happily infants of two and three months of age." (t. ii, p. 419.)

13

dered bleeding for an infant *three days old;* he caused his own wife to be bled eight times in the veins of the arm, and afterward bled her in those of the foot; she recovered, and he exclaimed: "*Vive!* the happy method of Galen, and the fine verse of Joachim de Bellay:

'O bonne, ô saincte, ô divine saignée!'

Now for cathartics. There is first a patient "who has been purged *thirty-two times* every other day;" there is another who has been bled, in all, *seventy-two* times, and purged *forty;* again, it is the doctrine of Galen and Hippocrates "to purge every day,—*quotidie licet purgare*," on condition, however, that senna is used: senna and phlebotomy are the whole of medicine.[1]

"We cure more patients," says Guy-Patin, "with a good lancet and a pound of senna, than the Arabians could with all their syrups and their opiates;" and his patients died, (for certainly all did not

(1) [Moliere must have had him in mind when writing his burlesque of the examination of an aspirant for a degree by the Faculty of Medicine in "*Le Malade imaginaire.*" To all questions in regard to the treatment of any disease the candidate duly responds

"Clysterium donare
Postea seignare
Ensuita purgare!"

And if this does not prove successful, the only course is to

"Reseignare, repurgare et reclysterisare!" —*Tr.*]

recover,) like those of the physician described by Boileau:

"L'un meurt vide de sang, l'autre plein de séné!"[1]

Guy-Patin started with the excellent principle of simplifying medicine and he ended by reducing it to bleeding and senna. A physician of our day, as resolute and as bold as Guy-Patin has reduced it to *leeches* and *gum-water*. In everything human there is some evil; in reform it is exaggeration.

It must not be thought, however, that Guy-Patin was always as unreasonable as in the extracts here given. No one had better sense, or was clearer and more judicious than he was at times. A wiser, better and more complete judgment upon the comparative merits of Greek and Arabian medicine has never been rendered than that which follows:

"As to the Arabians, I will tell you what I think; in regard to their doctrines, all they had valuable was taken from the Greeks; in regard to their remedies, they lived in a time when they could have had better ones than existed in the days of Hippocrates; but they abused them, and introduced that miserable arabesque pharmacy with a multitude of useless and superfluous drugs. The great abuse of medicine comes from a plurality of useless remedies and these caused blood-letting to be too much neglected. The Arabians are the

(1) *Art poetique*, chant. iv.

cause of both . . . . . Mesue has too much credit in the world . . . . . But we should be very wrong to abandon and give up good remedies which have been in use from the time of the Arabians, in order to return to those of the days of Hippocrates which are far less valuable . . . . . It is the doctrine of indications which has made the physician what he is; and for this we are entirely indebted to the Greeks."

In spite of his admiration of Hippocrates he admitted that there was one passage of that great man's works which, being misunderstood, "had cut the throat, and cost the life of more than fifty thousand persons." He says elsewhere, "It is a fine aphorism, but it should not be abused; our patients have nothing to do with our scholastic disputes."

Finally, even *antimony* obtains from him in calmer moments more circumspect remarks. "If any one is to make use of this remedy, which in its nature is so pernicious and so extremely dangerous, he should be a good theoretical and practical physician and very judicious, neither ignorant nor reckless; it is not a proper drug for the rattle-headed."

Nothing could be more judicious. New remedies, when they are energetic, demand a *judicious and experienced physician.* We should study them, watch them and follow them; not reject and proscribe them nor condemn them by *decrees of the*

Faculty.[1] In what condition should we have been now had our predecessors followed Guy-Patin and the Faculty? We should not have had antimony, opium, or cinchona; we should have known nothing of the circulation of the blood, the lymphatic vessels, the receptaculum chyli, and many other things; we should have been without both chemistry and physiology, the two sciences which have given us modern medicine. How could the dean of the faculty of medicine of Paris, a professor of the College of France, for Guy-Patin filled both these offices, how, we ask, could he write such words as the following, while standing side by side with the great Englishman, Harvey, who discovered the circulation of the blood, and the greatest of Frenchmen, Descartes, who proclaimed it?

"If M. Duryer knows only how to tell falsehoods and the circulation of the blood, he knows only two things, of which I heartily hate the first and care very little about the second. If he returns I will teach him more important things in medicine than the pretended circulation."[2]

(1) There were two decrees of the Faculty against antimony. [A sketch of the celebrated contest between the Galenical and chemical physicians, and a notice of the decrees and counter decrees in regard to antimony will be found in the "Revolutionary History of the Materia Medica," in Paris' Pharmacology.—*Tr.*]

(2) *Lettres*, t. i., p. 513. The *pretended circulation!*—Moliere could not do better. "But that which pleases me in him above

Pecquet was at Paris with Guy-Patin; perhaps he prescribed antimony; however, he discovered the reservoir of the chyle, the last fact which completed the new theory of the circulation of the blood, and Guy-Patin contented himself with saying: "The whole discovery of Pecquet is a novelty which I am quite ready to believe when it shall have been demonstrated, and when it proves of convenience and utility *in morborum curatione; quo excepto* I will have nothing to do with it."

I hasten to leave this puerile language and these culpable prejudices of Guy-Patin, and return to what he did more illustrious and more worthy our attention. He was truly a wise and learned man; full of Greek and Latin knowledge, a man of belles-lettres; he said himself, "learning and good sense are all."

He says, "I love only Galen and Hippocrates; I esteem Fernel, Duret, Hollier, Heurnius; our good friend Gaspard Hoffman does not displease me at all, *propter suam breviloquentiam* and for his criticism; *cœteris lubens abstineo.* I employ what spare time I have better elsewhere; the ma-

everything else, and in which he follows my example, is that he follows blindly the opinions of our seniors, and that he has never wished to understand nor has he examined the reasons and experiments in favor of the *pretended discoveries* of our times in regard to the circulation of the blood, and other doctrines of the same class."—(Moliere. *Le Malade imaginaire.*)

jority of modern authors contain nothing but repetitions."

He employed better "elsewhere" his spare time; and it is easy to divine what he meant by "elsewhere."

"I am guilty of no dissipation except in my study with my books. The late M. Pietre, an incomparable man in goodness as well as in science, was accustomed to say that he was guilty of dissipation only in reading Cicero and Seneca, but that he easily brought himself back again to duty by the perusal of Galen and Fernel."

This trait is charming. He had that elevated mind in which the love of letters is a passion. He wished to go to Germany to see his friend Hoffman: he went to Basle "to see there the tomb of the great Erasmus." He visited the tombs of the kings at St. Denis: "some tears escaped me before the monument of that great and good king Francis I., who founded our college of royal professors; I must confess my weakness to you, I even kissed it, and that of his father-in-law Louis XII., the father of his people, and the best king we have ever had in France." He brought his two sons to the tomb of Fernel. "One hundred and two years ago to-day, the sixteenth of April, died J. Fernel, a great and illustrious man, of whom the memory will last as long as the world, *aut saltem quamdiu honos habebitur bonis litteris;* he is interred in St. Jacques-de-la-Boucharie, near here. I often take my two sons there and exhort them to become like him." He esteemed Fernel so highly that he would *prefer to be descended from him than to be king*. "I am delighted that you love our Fernel so well; he is one of my saints, with Galen and the late M. Pietre. I should esteem it a greater glory to be descended from Fernel than to be king of Scotland, or a relation of the emperor of Constantinople. Fernel was good, wise and learned."

He had the gift of writing and relating good stories: "Yesterday about two o'clock, in the wood of Vincennes, four of his physicians, (Mazarin's), viz: Guenaut, Valot, Bayer, and Beda, altercated, and could not agree about the disease of which a patient was dying. Bayer said the spleen was mortified; Guinaut said it was the liver; Valot said it was the lungs, and there was water in the chest; and Beda maintained that it was an abscess of the mesentery, and that the pus had been discharged, he had seen it in the stools; and in this case he had seen what none of the others saw!—Are they not skillful men!"

Moliere could not have omitted such a comic scene,[1] nor St. Simon, the eloquent St. Simon, the

(1) "The physicians debated below as usual, and did not fail to disagree, some saying that the disease arose from the brain, some from the intestines, some from the spleen, some from the liver."—(*Le Medecin malgré lui.*)

following striking passage among many others: "We live in Paris as Juvenal says of Rome: *hic vivimus ambitiosâ pauperpate*, etc. I see nothing but vanity, misery and avarice, imposture and rascality. God has reserved us for a knavish and dangerous age; it will soon be of great consequence to be an honest man, so much has corruption been increased among all sorts of people for forty years past, by war, by two cardinals, who have been two great tyrants, and by the reign of partisans, who have devoured and exhausted France."

His mind presented many analogies with the mind of Rabelais, of Bayle and of Voltaire; he called Juvenal *his dear friend;* he painted Tacitus "that master man" in a remarkable manner: "Cornelius Tacitus, who was a breviary of State, and the premier, or grand master of the secrets of the cabinet, and whom even M. de Balzac has somewhere called the *ancient original of modern finesse.* Cardinal Richelieu read and practiced Tacitus closely; he was also a terrible man. Machiavelli is another instructor for such ministers of state, but he is only a diminutive Tacitus."

[Le Sage also gives a similar ridiculous scene in chap. iii. of Book iv. of Gil Blas, in which two of the "most eminent physicians of Madrid" could not agree as to whether the humors should be purged off before being concocted or not, and as to what Hippocrates taught on the subject.—*Tr.*]

Finally, he had noble and virtuous friends. That *society*, which he dreamed for another world, he chose for himself in this: "Socrates and another philosopher consoled themselves in dying that they would see in the other world honest men, philosophers, poets and physicians. I am of the same sentiment. If I can there meet Cicero, Virgil, Aristotle, Plato, Juvenal, Horace, Galen, Fernel, Simon and Nicolas Pietre, Moreau and Riolan, I shall not be in bad company; there is something in that to console me."

His friends were the learned Naude, Gassendi, Lamoignon, whose names it is sufficient to mention, and this same Riolan and Pietre whom he hoped to meet hereafter. "Monsieur, the first president, sends for me sometimes to dine with him; he makes grand cheer for me; but his hearty reception is worth more than all the rest. I have promised to dine with him every Sunday of this Lent, and after that we will make other arrangements according to the season. It is pleasant to visit him for he is the most learned of the long robe in France. He is very acute and very civil, and says, smiling, that we must not speak evil of the jesuits and the monks, but he is delighted when a *bon mot* escapes me against them."

How full of interest are all these details now! "I supped lately with M. the premier president, who sent to invite me in the morning. He complained because I did not call to see him, said that I ought sometimes to come and entertain him, and that I ought to have pity upon him on account of the difficulties he had in the administration of his office . . . . . After supper we entertained ourselves by the fireside. Among other things he told me I ought to be very happy, since having visited my patients I had only to pass my time with my books; that, for him, his office was killing him, and he thought himself far more unfortunate than M. Patin. In truth, great dignities are charges, which like hand-cuffs and fetters deprive us of our liberty and make us the slaves of all the world. This public office obliges him to give audience to every one, takes away from him the means and the leisure for diverting himself with study which he naturally loves, and obliges him to rise every palace day at four o'clock in the morning; yet nevertheless, and notwithstanding all his complaints, it is a very fine and a very important dignity." . . . . .

What a fine quaint style, how expressive, precise, and how well-marked by all the shades of life! And on the other hand, what a picture of this first president, who gets up at *four o'clock in the morning*, who has not leisure to *divert himself with study*, who says we *must not speak evil of the jesuits*, and who is *delighted* when others do it! All this is life-like.

I have said nothing yet of the character of Guy-Patin, and perhaps it is not necessary that I should. The friendship of the chief magistrate, and such an one as Lamoignon, is an index of this character. We have seen, too, the style of his writing. One of the qualities the most strongly marked of this style is the evidence it gives of the honest man.

I have just thrown a rapid glance upon Guy-Patin and his age: the age and the man both demand a closer examination, and this must be the object of another chapter.

VII.

GUY-PATIN AND THE FACULTY OF PARIS.

We have had until now only the *exterior* history of the Faculty of Medicine of Paris. Guy-Patin gives us its internal history. He exposes to us the hidden springs which moved this great body. He knows all its secrets, and keeps none of them. He tells us all because he does not know he is speaking for our benefit, and his account is the more reliable because he little thought he was writing history.

No one has better informed us in regard to the usages, or to speak like him, the *ceremonies*[1] of the Faculty. Let us commence with the most important act of this body, the election of dean. Guy-Patin was dean once, and three times his name remained in the hat. This is his account of the manner in which the affair was conducted:

"All the Faculty being assembled, the dean who is about to retire from office thanks the company for the honor which has been conferred upon him,

(1) "All these ceremonies are very ancient and are religiously observed, out of respect for their antiquity."—(T. ii., p. 566.)

and requests them to elect another to fill his place; the names of all the doctors present, for no absentee can be elected, are on the table on as many ballots; the first half, from above downward, are then placed in a hat, and this is called the *grand banc*. There are now one hundred and twelve members and the *grand banc* then consists of the first fifty-six. When these ballots have been well shaken and mixed in the hat by the *ancient*, or senior, of the company,[1] which is at present M. Riolan, the retiring dean draws out three, one after the other; and two names are also immediately drawn from the *petit banc*. Here are five doctors neither of whom can at this time be dean, but they are the electors, who, after having publicly taken an oath of fidelity, are shut in the chapel where they choose three members from the fellows present whom they judge worthy of the office—two being chosen from the *grand banc* and one from the *petit banc;* these three names are then placed in the hat by the ancient, and the dean, with widely extended arm draws one out, and the member whose name is drawn is the dean elect."

After the dean came the doctors-regent. They were elected in the same manner. And after these

(1) *L'ancien de la compagnie ou l'ancien maitre.* "The oldest doctor of the company is called the master and can not be termed dean; this being denied him by a decree of the court."—(T. ii., p. 566.)

followed the doctors, and for these the examinations were very numerous; there were some for the baccalaureate, for the license, and for the degree. There were theses of all kinds, the *quodlibetiares*, the *cardinal*, etc. They knew how to be severe, at least in the days of which I am speaking.

"Saturday, March 20th, we have passed ten bachelors who are about to commence their course of two years; we have also sent back two in order that they may amend and study better for the future; unless they do so within that period of time, they will fail of their duty, and we shall expel them from our schools as indolent and unworthy of our privileges."

I remark the two years of *perpetual disputation;* our two years of clinical instruction are assuredly much better spent, and yet we should exaggerate nothing; these practiced debaters often became admirable men of science. Says Riolan: "When the king, Henry the Great, wished to prove the falsehoods in the books of M. Plessis-Mornay in regard to religion, which the Bishop of Evreux, since Cardinal du Perron, promised to point out and verify, as he did, a learned physician of our school, named Martin, was chosen to oppose Casaubon who was held the most learned man of the age, after Joseph Scaliger who lived in Holland."[1]

(1) *Curieuses recherches sur les ecoles en medicine de Paris et de Montpellier.* Paris, 1651, p. 34.)

It was by their science, their erudition and their literary attainments that the Fernels, the Holliers, the Durets, and the two Riolans, father and son, elevated, ennobled, *emancipated*, if I may so speak, the science of medicine. It is their glory and it will be eternal. Medicine will never forget that to them she owes her lustre.

I return to the Faculty. Its intimate structure is plain enough. This body governed itself and recruited itself as it had formed itself. "Our school," says Riolan, "had for founders neither the kings of France nor the city of Paris from whom it has never received any assistance in money. It was founded and has been maintained at the expense of individual physicians, who have contributed to build it, to endow it, etc."[1]

The *corps medical* of Paris, taken in itself, was a little republic, a true republic, which had the doctors for citizens, the Faculty for a senate and the Dean for a chief. This chief was only elected for two years, but during that time he had a real authority. "He is," says Guy-Patin, "the master of the bachelors who are in their pupilage, he directs the discipline of the school, he keeps our registers which extend back more than five hundred years, he has the two seals of the Faculty, he receives our revenue and renders us an account of

(1) *Curieuses recherches*, etc., p. 29.

it, he signs and approves all the theses, he causes the doctors to preside according to their rank, he calls the Faculty together whenever he pleases, and without his consent it can not assemble except under a decree from the court which it is necessary to obtain; with the four examiners he conducts the rigorous examinations of a week's duration, he is one of the three deans who govern the University with the rector and is one of those who elect that officer; he has double the revenue of the others and that amounts sometimes to a very considerable sum; he has great responsibilities, much honor, and a large amount of business; he conducts the legal proceedings of the Faculty and speaks even in the grand chamber before the advocate general."[1] . . . .

Our little republic had within it all the good and all the evil of great ones. Its individual members were passionately devoted to the glory of the *corps*, and this was the good; but every moment saw the formation of parties, divisions, cabals and factions, and this was the evil. Often one party condemned the other; sometimes even *expelled* them. In 1651, Guenaut, Beda and Cornuti, who had *allowed themselves to be carried away by antimony*,[2] were condemned by the Faculty: "this made them return

(1) *Lettres de Gui-Patin*, t. ii., p. 565.

(2) Expression of Gui-Patin.

to their duty," says Guy-Patin, "and if hereafter they are wanting, we shall not be; the law and the efficacy of the decree will be applied to them so efficaciously, that they will remain exiled."[1] Often one party reversed what the other had done. In 1566, one party obtained the issue of a decree against antimony,[2] and in 1666, just a century later, another party passed a directly contrary decree in favor of the remedy.

When we see the Faculty thus founding itself, maintaining itself, endowing itself, and owing everything to its members and nothing to the state, one can well understand that *independence* which was so peculiar to it, of which it was so jealous, and which the state always respected. Our kings treated with the Faculty. Louis XI. wished to have a manuscript of Rhazes copied, which the Faculty owned; but the Faculty would not lend the manuscript to the royal applicant until he had deposited security.[3] Richelieu exerted his influence in favor of the admission to the doctorate of the sons of the *gazetier* Renaudot, a man most violently hated by the Faculty; he persisted, the Faculty resisted, and Richelieu was obliged to abandon his point. "All individual men die," says Guy-Patin proudly, "but companies never die.

(1) *Lettres de Gui-Patin*, t. ii., p. 587.

(2) There was another decree against antimony, in 1615.

(3) T. i., p. 37. Note of M. Reveillé-Parise.

The most powerful man in Europe for a hundred years, except crowned heads, was Cardinal Richelieu. He made the whole earth tremble; he made Rome itself fear him; he shook the King of Spain on his throne; nevertheless he was not able to make our company receive the two sons of the gazetier, who were licentiates, but who will not for a long time become doctors."

Finally, the Faculty perished like all associated bodies, all republics, by the exaggeration of its peculiar principles. Its grand aim had been to restore *Greek* and *Latin* medicine. This attained it stopped obstinately and fatally. It advanced no farther; but everything around was advancing. Modern chemistry, anatomy and physiology were discovered. These sciences the Faculty proscribed. When the government earnestly wished to extend a knowledge of them it was obliged to have them taught elsewhere. The *Jardin du Roi* was created, or restored. The Faculty proscribed chemistry and this, it said, *for good causes and considerations;*[1] in the garden it was taught by a chair established expressly for that purpose. Riolan,[2] the first anato-

(1) Expressions of the Faculty in its *Remonstrances* upon the creation of the Jardin du Roi. See the *Notices historique sur le Museum d'histoire naturelle* par Laurent de Jussieu: *Annales du Museum d'hist. nat.*, t. i., p. 12.

(2) It is curious that Riolan, who rejected modern anatomy on behalf of the Faculty and would have excluded it from the garden, was one of the first who felt the need of such a gar-

mist in the ranks of the Faculty, rejected the circulation of the blood, the lymphatic vessels, the receptaculum chyli, etc.; they were taught in the garden by Dionis. Dionis tells us himself, in his epistle to the king (Louis XIV.) "It is there that the circulation of the blood and the new discoveries have happily freed us from those errors, which we scarcely dared to leave, and which the authority of the ancients so long fixed upon us."[1]

Dionis afterward tells us that "this establishment, although most useful for the public, did not fail to find opposition, which was raised on the part of those who pretended that they alone had the right to teach and demonstrate anatomy."[2]

den. It is an honor which should not be forgotten, although he had so many other claims upon our memory. "You can likewise inform the king," he says in the dedicatory epistle of his *Gigantologie*, addressed to the Duc de Luynes, "you can inform the king, who only desires the health and preservation of his subjects, of the necessity of a royal garden in the University of Paris, such as Henry the Great had laid out for Montpellier; which, if we obtain from the king, by your intercession, you will oblige all France, which will appreciate the great benefit you will have procured for all those who practice medicine."—(p. 8.)

(1) *L'anatomie de l'homme suivant la circulation du sang et les nouvelles decouvertes, demontrée au Jardin du roi, Paris*, 1716: *Epitre au roi*, p. 2.

(2) *Ibid*, Preface, p. 6.—Modern anatomy finally passed from the garden to the Faculty: often the same professor taught it in both places. See Winslow and others.

It may readily be surmised who those were who "formed opposition," and who "pretended that they alone had the right to teach and demonstrate anatomy." They were the same persons who pursued the surgeons and the apothecaries with unpitying and incessant hostility. In truth, the Faculty did not pretend to reject surgery as it had rejected the new sciences, but it excluded the surgeons. Guy-Patin spoke of the surgeons in terms which causes us to blush for him. The government was obliged to do for surgery what it had already done for the new sciences. The Faculty closed their doors against it, the government opened others for it. The Royal College of Surgery was created. "This latter title (the title of the Faculty,)" said La Martiniere to King Louis XV, "was the object of our ambition, but, since your supreme will has deigned to accord us the title of *College royal*, the honor of depending immediately upon your Majesty suffices to console us for every other distinction."[1] The Academy of Surgery appeared, and appeared with an *eclat* which attracted the attention of all Europe. The first volume of the *Memoirs* of this Academy is the most beautiful monument of French surgery. The Royal Society of Medicine came in its turn, and then this ancient Faculty, which had

(1) *Memoire présenté au roi par son premier chirurgien Lamartiniere*, etc.

lasted eight centuries,[1] terminated its existence. After the revolution of 1789, when the department of public instruction was reörganized, the remaining members of the Royal Society of Medicine served as the nucleus of the new Faculty.

Guy-Patin tells us everything about his Faculty, not only that which is serious but that which is the reverse. I have just described some of the ceremonies of the Faculty. Each of these events was followed by a *feast:* "Saturday, March 20th, we received six bachelors . . . . . The same day an entertainment was given to the schools." Then Guy-Patin enumerates all the invited, carefully indicating the rank of each: "the dean and censors, the ancient deans, the four examiners, the five doctors, the four seniors of the schools, the ordinary professors, some friends of the dean, who are the best men of the schools and the most considerable of the Faculty . . . . . I never saw such enjoyment on the part of all; there was nothing but merriment and good cheer."

He was elected dean on the 4th of November, 1650, and on the 1st of December, he *gave his entertainment.* "Having returned home this morning, I found your letter there, which has increased the joy I had yesterday in giving my feast on

(1) "By the perusal of ancient books," says Riolan, "we can show proof of more than six hundred years."—(*Curieuses recherches*, etc., p. 28.) Riolan wrote this in 1651.

account of my election. Thirty-six of my colleagues made merry; I never saw so much drinking and laughing by steady people, and even by our seniors: they had the best old wine of Bourgogne which I reserved for the feast. I received them in my room, where, besides the tapistry, are the portraits of Erasmus, the two Scaligers, father and son, Casaubon, Muret, Montaigne, Charron, Grotius, Heinsius, Saumaise, Fernel, de Thou, and our good friend Gabriel Naudé, librarian of Mazarin, which is only his external quality, for of the internal ones he has as many as any one can have; he is very learned, good, and wise, has gained experience and is cured of the folly of the age, a faithful and constant friend for thirty-two years. There were also three other portraits of excellent men—of the late M. de Sales, bishop of Geneva, of Justus Lipsius, and finally of Francois Rabelais. What do you say of this assembly? Were not my guests in good company?"

Everything is worthy of note in this recital; the *joy* of Guy-Patin, the *old wine*, the *seniors* who *laughed* and who *drank*, and above them the portraits of Erasmus, Casaubon, Montaigne, Rabelais, Fernel, and other worthies, with the friend Naudé, Mazarin's librarian, *which is only his external quality!* And how completely all this is characteristic of Guy-Patin! the friendly, the erudite, the critical, the enthusiastic, the malicious, the good-natured, and finally the spiritual, bold, and *déniaisé* Guy-Patin!

Guy-Patin is inexhaustible when he speaks of the Faculty; he is, if possible, still more so when speaking of men. It is first Riolan,[1] his master, his friend, who took him for his assistant,[2] who designed him for his successor at the Royal College of France, whom Guy-Patin calls *our master in everything;* "and of the men of the world who knew most of particulars and of curiosities, not only in medicine but also in history . . . . . at once a very good man, and naturally very sarcastic, ... who would that all the world wrote against him,

(1) It is scarcely necessary to state that *Riolan* of whom I speak in this chapter, is Riolan the son, born in 1580 and died in 1657. He alone was a contemporary of Guy-Patin as Riolan the senior was born in 1539 and died in 1605.

(2) Here is something curious in regard to the college of France. "M. Moreau will not give up his place as Royal professor to his son until death, because, as he is one of the seniors of the College he has far greater receipts, on account of augmentation in favor of the earliest received, than his son, who being one of the youngest, will only receive six hundred livres, while the father receives one thousand, or nearly eleven hundred livres. Morin, the mathematician who is immediately next to him has the entire sum, four hundred crowns, the same as the dean M. Riolan; when the latter dies I shall take his place, having the same reversion as the youngest Moreau, and then I enter upon the receipt of six hundred livres; afterward I succeed and increase as others die who were received before me."—(T. ii., p. 162.)

. . . . . . keeping himself close in his study, with a stove for warmth in the manner of the Germans, and there writing against antimony, ... drinking wine all day, or adding to it but very little water, and saying for excuse, that it was old wine of Bourgogne."

Then it is the family of the Pietres, all *incomparable*, the elder above all, for he presided as dean when antimony was proscribed: *in cujus decanatu latum est decretum adversus stibium*, says Guy-Patin.

With Guy-Patin there is no one of medium quality; he is is either *incomparable* or *abominable*, according as he opposes antimony or not! For example, Guenaut, "wicked charlatan, obstinate in all things . . . . . playing the tyrant in our schools, abusing at the expense of the public, the iniquity and impunity of the age . . . . . a brazen-faced prescriber of antimony, *peste antimoniale*," etc., etc. Guenaut was not probably all that, although he must have been very lively, very active, very much occupied, and a man of some station, for Boileau reckons him among the *embarrassments* of the streets of Paris:

> "Guenaut sur son cheval en passant m'eclabousse."[1]

Vautier is "wicked, very boastful and very ignorant; the first physician of the king and the

(1) *Satire* vi.

last of the kingdom in capacity;" and you immediately divine why: *he gives antimony;* and that is not all, *he speaks ill of senna and bleeding!* "M. Vautier slanders our Faculty frequently and we know it well; he says that we use nothing but senna and depletion; he has given antimony very boldly."

M. Morisset, on the contrary, does not give antimony; see what different language! "Le sieur Morisset is sixty-seven years old, ... he has a good appearance; he seems to be boastful, but is not so; he has, however, what might render him so more than others, for he is a very learned and skillful man. He converses well, he speaks eloquently, he consults with judgment, speaks Latin well, understands Greek, and would never prescribe antimony." He would never prescribe *antimony:* "even although he has been implored to do so, and principally by Guenaut."[1]

Guy-Patin is passionate in everything: in politics as well as in medicine. In medicine, what he hated most was *antimony* and *Guenaut*, in politics it was the *Jesuits* and *Mazarin.* He did not like Richelieu any better. "Cardinal Richelieu," he says, "resembled Tiberius, ... he is a splenetic, who wished to reign . . . . . Mazarin did not love vengeance or blood, but he was a great cut-purse."

(1) *Lettres de Gui-Patin*, t. iii., p. 412.

It often happened that he treated the Jesuits, the monks, and the Pope himself, as *if they had given antimony!* On the contrary he showed a marked affection for Parliament, for liberty, for every kind of independence, political, civil and religious, for the Fronde, for Cardinal de Retz. "The diet of Ratisbon is also spoken of, and it is said that the king will send M. le Cardinal de Retz there. Would to God that he be reinstated in favor! he is a man of spirit, who loves glory and the public honor, to which he will infallibly be of benefit." And as soon as he saw Louis XIV., then quite young, he foresaw in the young prince the great king: he says, "the king is a prince well-proportioned, large and tall, not yet twenty years old. He is," he continues, "a prince worthy of being loved even by those to whom he has never been of service, who has great thoughts, and upon whose inclinations France will be able to found a repose of which Richelieu and Mazarin have deprived her. I feel a violent attachment for him."

I finish with regret; for it is difficult to quit Guy-Patin, a man so singular of his class: writer, physician, scholar, devout worshiper of the ancients, a passionate opponent of the moderns, *a spirit all fire*, as he says himself, and joining to these, pure morals, warm and constant friendship, and the liveliest tenderness for his children: "I love children dearly," he says; "I have six, and it seems to me that I have not enough; I am very happy to learn that you have a little daughter; we have only one and she is so gentle and so agreeable that we love her almost as much as we do our five boys." . . . . .

We know that he was not a happy father. Of his six children, five died young, a loss which brought from his pen these touching words: *quodam modo moritur ille qui amittit suos.* His eldest son, Robert, for whom he had obtained the succession of his chair in the College of France, died early; and his deeply-loved son Charles, his "*dear Carolus*," as he always called him, the illustrious son who inherited his father's genius and his passion for study, was exiled.

As to himself, he was born[1] on the 31st of August, 1601, and died on the 30th of August, 1672. His *Letters* commence in 1630 and end in the year of his death. They are addressed, by turns, to two physicians of Troyes, the two Berlins, father and son, and to two physicians of Lyons, Charles Spon and Andre Falconet.

M. Reveillé-Parise alludes to some small works by Guy-Patin:[2] these works are very insignificant.

(1) At La Place, a little hamlet of the commune of Hodenc-en-Bray (not far from Beauvais,) an ancient province of Picardy.

(2) In his *Notice biographique* preceding his edition of the *Lettres de Guy-Patin.*

Guy-Patin, in truth, wrote nothing but his *Letters;* and these letters, in spite of a boldness of thought often excessive,[1] in spite of language often too violent, in spite of many errors in facts and many prejudices against men, these letters, the brilliant expression of a superior mind and a fiery spirit will ensure his remembrance, for he has put that in them which never dies—style.

Guy-Patin is the most spiritual and witty physician who ever wrote, if we except Rabelais, of whom, however, physician was only the "*external quality.*"

[PARIS alludes to one of them in the "Revolutionary History of the Materia Medica" prefixed to his Pharmacologia. It was entitled "*Antimonial Martyrology*" and consisted of a register of unsuccessful cases in which antimony had been given!—*Tr.*]

(3) "He wrote to one of his friends with a liberty not only entire, but sometimes excessive; elogiums are not very common in his *Lettres* and what predominates there is very independent philosophic spleen."—(Fontenelle: *Eloge de Dodart.*)

TABLE OF CONTENTS.

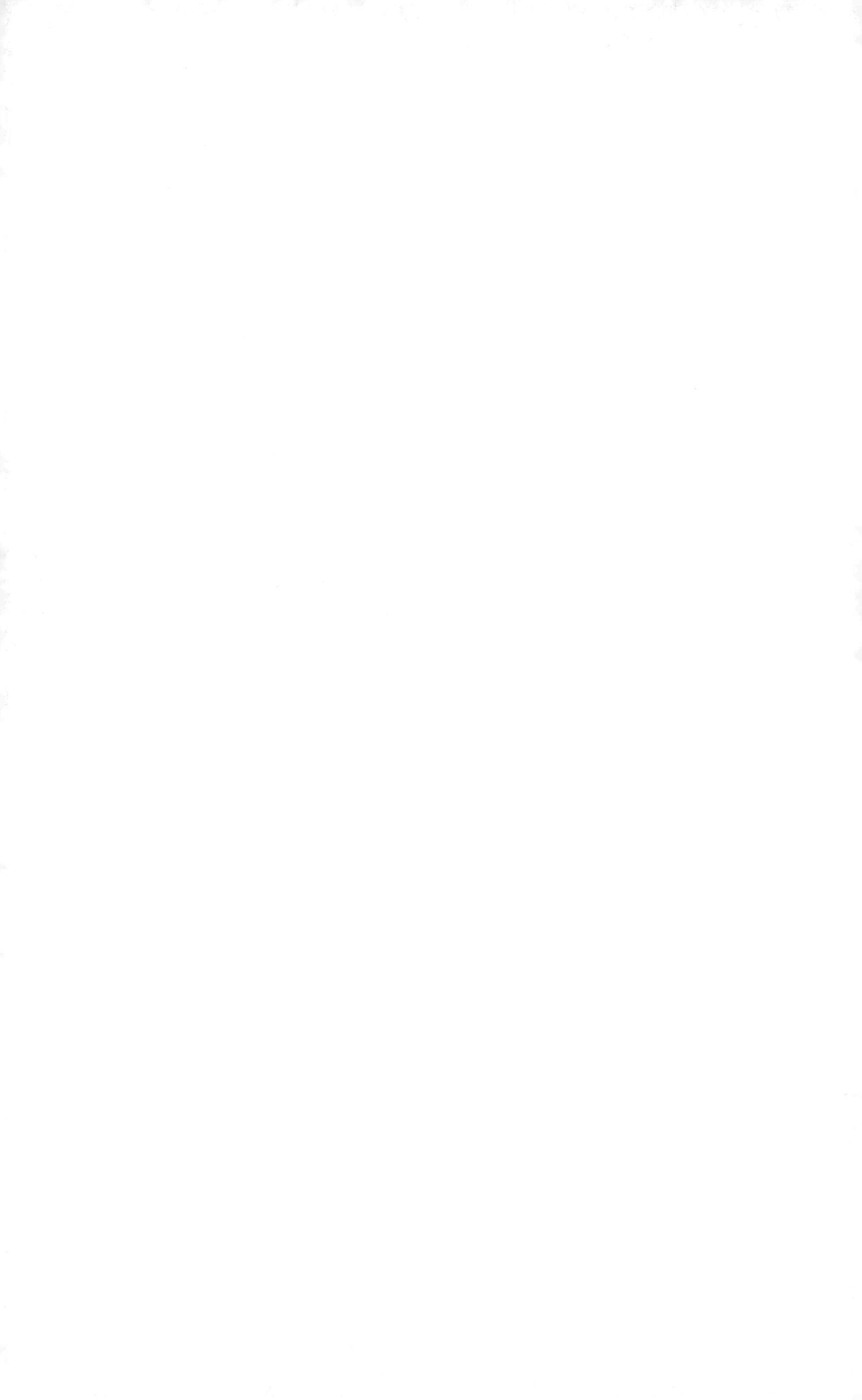

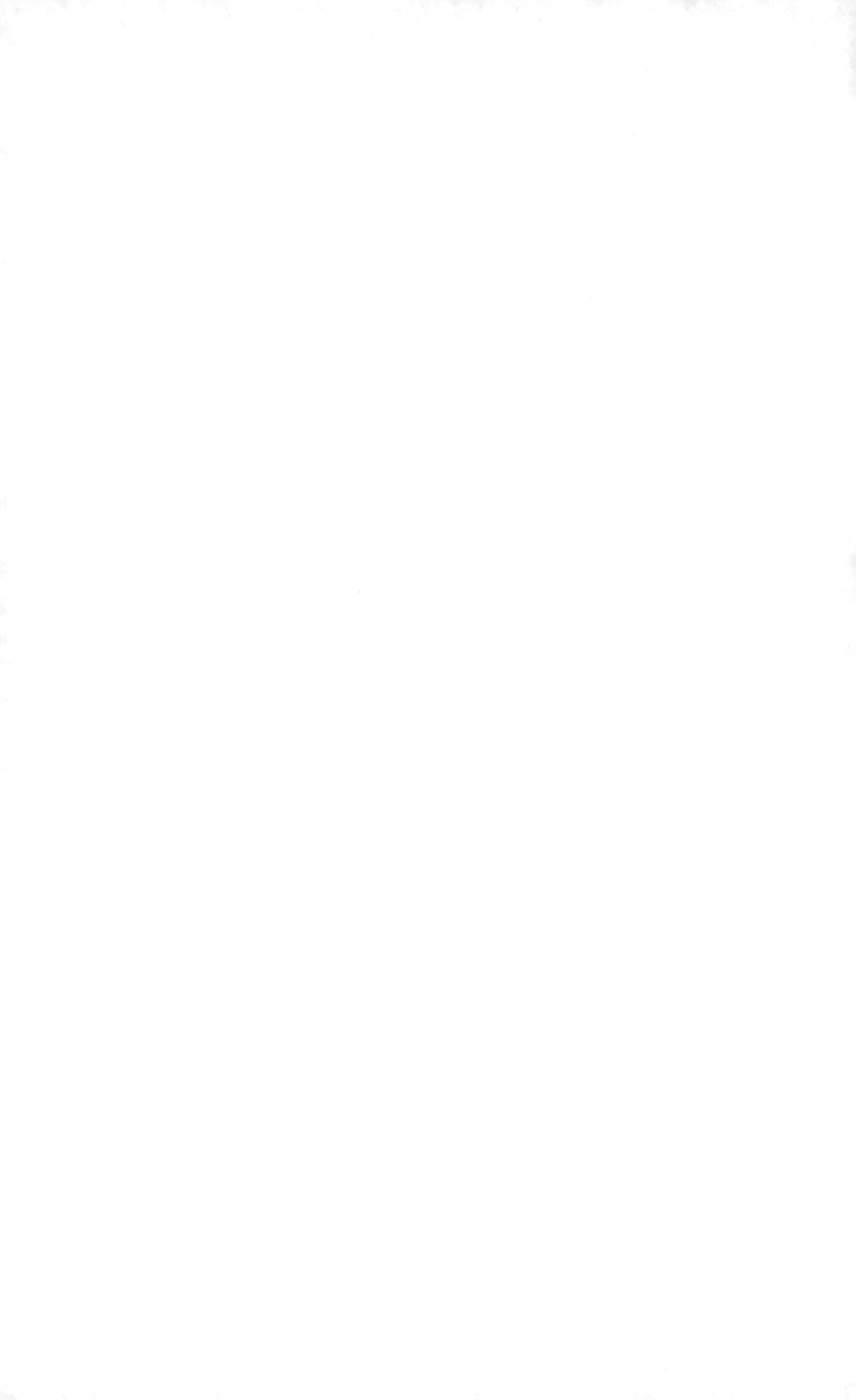

www.ingramcontent.com/pod-product-compliance
Lightning Source LLC
LaVergne TN
LVHW011236110826
845150LV00006B/1655

* 9 7 8 1 4 2 5 5 1 4 3 1 0 *